HEALTH AND THE DIVISION OF LABOUR

HEALTH AND THE DIVISION OF LABOUR

Edited by

MARGARET STACEY, MARGARET REID, CHRISTIAN HEATH and ROBERT DINGWALL

CROOM HELM
London

PRODIST
New York

Croom Helm Ltd, 2-10 St John's Road, London SW11

British Library Cataloguing in Publication Data

Sociology, Health and Illness (Conference), 1976
Health and the division of labour.
1. Medical personnel – Congresses 2. Division of labour – Congresses
I. Title II. Stacey, Margaret
301. 5'5 RA410.6

ISBN 0-85664-487-0

First published in the United States by
PRODIST
a division of
Neale Watson Academic Publications, Inc.
156 Fifth Avenue, New York 10010

Library of Congress Cataloging in Publication Data

Main entry under title:

Health and the division of labour.

1. Medical personnel – Addresses, essays, lectures.
2. Social medicine – Addresses, essays, lectures.
I. Stacey, Margaret. [DNLM: 1. Health occupations.
2. Health services. 3. Sociology. W21 H432]
RA410.6.H4 331.7'61'3621 77-8198
ISBN 0-88202-119-2 (Prodist)

Printed in Great Britain by Biddles Ltd, Guildford, Surrey

CONTENTS

INTRODUCTION

The papers in this volume are all drawn from the 1976 British Sociological Association Conference, organised around the theme of health and illness. The many papers given at the Conference reflect the increasing range of research carried out in this field. One collection of papers has already been published in a companion volume *Health Care and Health Knowledge*. It deals with the production and maintenance of medical knowledge and medical policy. This second volume represents another line of interest in health and illness, that is, studies of occupations within the field. The papers focus particularly upon themes of occupational control and the relationships which exist between the various groups which interact in this context.

The sociology of occupations has typically concentrated its attention on the high status occupations – the 'professions'. Initial thinking, now largely abandoned as unproductive, sought to list the ingredients which gave certain groups the qualities of a profession. Traditional debates were challenged, however, and the field has diversified to encompass several perspectives and many debates. In the 1950s, for example, sociologists (especially those of the Chicago school) abandoned the search for 'professional' characteristics and turned instead to a consideration of the implications of being seen as a profession. Thus for the first time questions about *intra*professional relationships were raised, and problems about intergroup conflict studied, issues which still find a place in the writings of today. Sociologists also noted the wider resources of power available to professional groups through their license and mandate, a line of thinking which was steadily developed through to the work of Freidson, a welcome contributor to this volume.

Through his identification of autonomy as a critical determinant of professionalism, and his emphasis on the importance of indeterminacy of professional expertise, Freidson's work represents a powerful influence on current research. While Freidson elaborated the peculiar institutional control granted professional groups, others, notably Johnson (1972), extended the idea of professionalism as social control to examine the form such control might take and the conditions under which it may flourish.

Paralleling the study of professional groups has been an increased interest in unionisation of lower status groups as an alternative form of social control. For example some, particularly those of a Marxist tendency, have examined the organisation of the proletariat of the health services rather than the petit bourgeousie – readers will find examples of these studies in the following papers.

The development of pluralist theories of professionalisation has led to a broadening of interest in the sociology of occupations, and a more fruitful linking of theory to empirical research. At the same time, it raises problems for any student in the field, for little attempt is made to provide the study of occupations with a general (i.e. overarching) theory of professionalisation. This point is well illustrated in Friedson's paper, which acts as a general introduction to the other papers. Freidson presents a systematic analysis of the differing usages of the term 'profession' outlining the deficiencies of each usage and discussing the future which each implies for that branch of the labour market. The author offers no solutions as to which prediction may be the most accurate, for, as he argues, two analyses of the possible futures of professions may both be logical and yet at the same time contradictory.

Freidson's paper alerts the reader to the complexities (and confusions) of the rhetoric of this particular field of study. However, the underlying theme of the book, that of occupational control, negotiation and change, serves to unite the more substantive papers of this collection. Following Freidson, the next four papers offer contemporary analyses of the medical profession. Interestingly, the first two (non-British) papers very consciously locate the medical care system within the wider political context of their country. De Miguel describes the role and function of the medical profession as diffusers of the Spanish authoritarian political regime, arguing that within a non-democratic régime the professions are not oriented towards public 'need' but are placed in a position (which they hold not unwillingly) of being strongly influenced by the government, wherein the major policy decisions are made. The lack of autonomy of the profession in Spain is emphasised by studying the medical ideology, which reflects the moral tenets of the ruling régime. The context in which medical care is practised also plays an important part in the next paper from the United States. Gallagher outlines their *laissez-faire* system in which members of the medical profession maintain a basically economic relationship with their clients. A pull exists, however, between the avowedly egalitarian society and the obvious social inequalities, a tension which, in the health service, has resulted in certain illness conditions being nominated as policy diseases, deserving separate state that the social organisation of health is never fixed but remains fluid and open. Within the medical profession, for example, the superior status afforded hospital personnel is being challenged by the growing emphasis placed, possibly through economic necessity, on community practice and the general practitioner responsible for care in this context. Women, too, it seems likely, will play a more competitive part in the medical labour market of the future, despite efforts to maintain the *status quo*.

At the beginning of the volume Professor Freidson raised the important question of the future of these high status professional groups, of which medicine is taken to be an archetypical example. One answer implicit in many of the writings in this collection is that the continuing dominance of professions is not assured. Social and economic influences are ever liable to change the balance of power, so that other groups, possibly those now termed 'ancillary' to medicine, may gain greater control over their work. The division of labour within this area of health and illness, is, then, to repeat the central theme of the volume, always open to conflict, negotiation and change.

References

Johnson, T.J. (1971). *Professions and Power*, London, Macmillan.

THE FUTURES OF PROFESSIONALISATION[1]

Eliot Freidson

Until very recently, it was common for some of the most notable scholars of the day to emphasise the importance of professions in modern society, and to consider professionalisation to be a major social movement, transforming both society and the nature of work. Before the turn of the century, Spencer expatiated on the way in which professions augmented human life (Spencer, 1896). Almost sixty years ago the Webbs discussed professional associations as one form of 'Associations of Producers' (in contrast to associations of consumers) which might provide a viable alternative to capitalistic forms of productive organisation (Webb and Webb, 1917). Shortly afterwards, R.H. Tawney (1920: 91-122) urged the nationalisation of British industry so as to 'professionalise' it, with all workers assuming responsibility for the quality of their work. In a rather different political context, Carr-Saunders (1928) pointed to the growth of professionalism as a hopeful sign of the times and in his later work, with P.A. Wilson (Carr-Saunders and Wilson, 1933: 493-494) he predicted the extension of professionalism 'upwards and outwards', and the slower but continuous extension 'downwards' to transform routine intellectual and manual occupations. Subsequently, T.H. Marshall (1939: 325-340) noted modern society's increasing demand for professionalised services, the increasing number and type of professionals, and their changing relationship to the welfare state. By our day, Parsons (1968: 545) could say that 'the massive emergence of the professional complex . . . is the crucial structural development in twentieth-century society', and Bell (1976: 144) could predict that in the emerging post-industrial society of the future, 'professionals will be a major feature'.

With some few and recent exceptions to be discussed later in this paper, there seems to be rather remarkable unanimity about professions – agreement, first, that they represent a distinct kind of occupation which is of special importance to the effective and humane functioning of modern society, second, that they have been growing in number and importance throughout this century, and, third, that they will increase in number and importance in the future, into the next century. But in a very curious way we are left in limbo by such assessments and predictions, for they do not provide us with the intellectual tools by which we can connect them to concrete occupations. Indeed, when one examines such work closely, one finds sufficient confusion and contradiction in the use of the word, 'profession', and related words like 'professionalism' and 'professionalisation' that one cannot be at all sure that Parsons, for example, refers to the same occupations as Marshall in his formulation, or that Bell refers to the same as Hughes (1971). If that is indeed the case, then the unanimity is more apparent than real, relying more on common use of the same *word* than on common agreement about what the word refers to. Thus, they may very well be at once talking to each other in general and talking past each other in particular. This makes it singularly difficult for any genuine debate to take place, and seriously handicaps the systematic accumulation of information and the refinement and elaboration of concepts characteristic of true scholarship.

We all know that there are many usages and definitions connected with the term, 'profession'. (For one review of definitions, see Millerson, 1964: 1-9.) Part of the confusion stems from the fact that people are often prone to use the word as a means of flattering themselves and others (cf. Becker, 1970: 87-103). Another source of confusion lies in the fact that the word is used to refer both to concrete historical occupations and to an intellectual construct or ideal type, without consistent attention to the relationship between the two. And finally, an often unrecognised source of confusion lies in the fact that some analysts employ the term to characterise a broad social stratum including many occupations, while others use it to characterise particular occupations. Indeed, the word may be so hopelessly corrupted that its use is a positive handicap to the development of systematic concepts for the study of work and its organisation (cf. Habenstein, 1963: 291-300). No matter what one may wish, the problem cannot be solved by banning the use of the word: it is too well entrenched in the language of too many to be dropped out of sociological usage. Nor can the problem be solved by legislating academic usage: even if the power to legislate and enforce usage existed, there is no generally agreed conceptual rationale to justify dictating one usage rather than another. We are on our own, for better or for worse. What can be done? How can we assess the future of professionalisation?

It may be that our difficulties can be at least tempered by a more considered approach to the issues of usage – that is, by being more aware of how referents change from one usage to another, and what the implications of different usages are for what we are trying to talk about. This is not to suggest that any solution lies in mere review of various definitions, for the reviews of the past do not seem to have helped much. They have not helped much, I believe, because they have attempted to review and then adjudicate the importance of all of the traits or attributes imputed to professions, treating those attributes as additive rather than parts of a system (cf. Johnson, 1972: 23ff.). Past concern has been more with the precise traits by which to characterise a profession than with close examination of the empirical referents and theoretical implications of any single trait, and the relation of one trait to another. The issues involved in the concept of profession, I believe, can be better clarified by examining one variable or attribute at a time, particularly those implied by some of the most common denotations of the word. Taken one at a time, they can also be used by extrapolation from their past and present distribution to trace the future of professions and professionalisation. This is what I shall do here, hoping both to clarify the implications of various definitions and usages, and to facilitate the task of making sense of the contradictory readings of the future of professionalisation.

Because professions do not exist in isolation from other occupations, it seems appropriate to begin the discussion with the broadest usage of the term, a usage which in essence defines both what is *bona fide* work, and who is a *bona fide* worker: it defines the boundaries of the labour force itself. Following that discussion, I will discuss attempts to define professions as a particular stratum of the labour force. The ambiguities of that definition will then lead me to discuss professions as special kinds of status groups – as organisations of workers who have gained a monopoly over the right to control their own labour. The discussion of profession as occupational monopoly will then be used as the conceptual resource by which to make sense of social psychological conceptions of professions as being composed of workers who are somehow especially dedicated or committed. Finally, I shall conclude by reassessing both the problem of defining and studying professions and the problem of predicting their future.

The Future of Market-Related Labour

The broadest and most general use of the word 'profession' is built upon the distinction between 'professional' and 'amateur'. In that contrast, one can see the 'amateur' as one who performs a given set of tasks without conscious and calculating concern for their exchange value in the market, and the 'professional' as one who performs them in a contracted market exchange by which he gains his living. In that usage, the word 'profession' is a synonym of both 'occupation' and 'vocation' in

English, and corresponds to the general usage of *Beruf* in German[2] and *profession* in French. Performing market-related labour for one's living is one's professional vocation, while performing labour unconnected with a market is one's amateur avocation.

Simplistic and primitive as it may seem, the distinction is one that establishes relatively clear boundaries between (a) what is to be defined as work or labour and what is not, and (b) who is to be defined as a *bona fide* worker and who not. Essentially, it defines work or labour as any regular activity with an exchange value. Neither the intrinsic character of the activity itself, nor the skill its performance requires, nor the physical exertion expended during its performance is salient to distinguishing professional from amateur or work from non-work. Nor does the social role involved in the activity (cf. Hall, 1975, 3-7) discriminate professional from amateur. The same activity, involving the same social relations among performers, can be undertaken by either professional or amateur. What makes the activity 'work' is its exchange value. What makes a performer a 'worker' or a 'professional' is his relationship to the market. Activities not undertaken in the context of the market may not therefore be defined as work by this definition, nor may those who perform for the intrinsic pleasure of performance or for the admiration and gratitude of others be defined as 'professionals' or as 'workers'.

This lay distinction between professional and amateur, employing participation in the labour market as its essential criterion, also constitutes, at bottom, the foundation for official delineations of the labour force or the working force in most advanced industrial societies (Jaffe, 1968: 469-474). In this sense, one meaning of 'professionalisation' may be said to be the process by which increasing proportions of the population come to be part of the officially defined labour force — the process by which fewer and fewer members of a population come to perform activities for the pleasure derived from their performance, for the benefit it provides others, or for the gratitude or admiration of others, and more and more come to perform them for the income it provides. Certainly there is little doubt about the very broad past trend of increase in such professionalisation as capitalism has transformed the world. A large number of tasks which were originally performed on a voluntary basis by amateurs or performed for personal or household use rather than for a market are now performed by full-time workers who gain their living thereby. Thus, the trend has been toward the professionalisation of tasks (cf. Mincer, 1968).

But can we project that trend into the future and forecast still more professionalisation? That question is very difficult to answer, for past changes have been by no means unilinear. First, we might remember that many women and children were members of the labour force in the nineteenth century, but were later removed from factory jobs and sent back to the household or to newly constituted schools. Historically, women are *returning* to the officially defined labour force. Second, we might remember that a significant proportion of the population in such countries as the United States has in effect dropped or been dropped out of the labour force, to be underemployed or unemployed wards of the welfare state – a status that is neither amateur nor professional. Third, we must remember that as the cost of labour has increased in most industrial countries, a number of activities that were once performed by market-related labour have been reverting back to the amateur. In some cases, economic necessity alone has motivated people to do-it-themselves; in others, a distinct ideology of self-help has encouraged people to do their own work (if we can call it work when it is technically an avocation).

The trends, in short, are very complex. What we can say of the future cannot be predicated realistically on any simple notion that one can take a finite universe of tasks and project a trend of their 'professionalisation'. Some tasks will disappear entirely, others will be merged into new combinations, others will be returned to amateurs working alone or with others, and still others will leave the hands of amateurs and be professionalised. On balance, it does not seem to me that one can make any prophecy based on a quantitative trend toward more or less market-related labour in the future, if only because of the analytical difficulties inherent in the criterion of market relations, difficulties compounded by non-market factors introduced by the welfare state and state socialism.

Diagnostic evidence of the limitations of the concept of market-related labour may be found in the contemporary cases of two large groups of people who perform often arduous tasks of generally recognised social value, but who neither enter the labour market in order to perform those tasks, nor enter into an economic exchange relationship with another as a condition for performing those tasks. I refer to housewives and to volunteer workers. In the strict sense of the distinction I have been discussing here, such persons are not working when they perform their tasks, nor are they to be identified as members of the labour force. They are amateurs rather than professionals, and while they may occupy themselves and identify themselves by such tasks, their tasks may not be used to delineate their occupations.[3]

This is not the place for extended discussion of either of these groups of people. Certainly the case of the housewife has been receiving a great deal of attention lately, and the anomalies and inequities of her position should be familiar to most by now (cf. Oakley, 1974). It is clear that she 'works' but is not identified as a worker, and that her tasks have great use-value but no market-value in the household in which they are performed. Her tasks may not be called hobbies, nor may they be said to be leisure pursuits. They do involve productive as well as consumption functions, but by market criteria neither are they work nor may she be said to be employed, to have an occupation or profession.

An equal, perhaps even greater challenge to the utility of a market definition of labour for sociological analysis may be found in the case of unpaid work taking place outside of the household – what is sometimes called volunteer work. In the case of volunteers, there is no need for identifying their activity as an occupation, because most of those performing volunteer tasks do so in their leisure time, and if not retired are otherwise engaged in market-related labour by which their occupations may be identified. The problem is how to identify their tasks as productive labour rather than as play or leisure. There is little doubt of the social productivity of much volunteer work. In the People's Republic of China, for example, unpaid labour mobilised and supervised by technical and political 'professional' cadres has accomplished remarkable feats of public sanitation (cf. Horn, 1969). For a number of reasons, not the least among them the difficulty of financing the expansion and maintenance of public services and facilities in both capitalist and state socialist nations, such volunteer labour might remain important and even grow in the future. Whatever else, it is a constant challenge to the practice of delineating both work and profession by their relation to the market. Let us hope that the sociology of the future can meet that challenge by developing less arbitrary and more analytically satisfying criteria for distinguishing work from task, vocation from avocation and professional from amateur. Such criteria will be difficult to develop, for limited as it may be, the market criterion is parsimonious, is measured relatively easily, and refers to a phenomenon of undoubted importance.

The Future of the Professional Stratum of Labour

The amateur-professional distinction defines the general categories, 'work' and 'occupation'. Beyond setting those broad boundaries, it cannot discriminate among types of work or types of occupations. Most sociological literature takes the market definition of work and of occupation as given and then proceeds to discriminate types of work and occupation within the officially defined labour force. Very common in the macro-sociological literature is reference to a specific 'class' of professionals as a stratum of the labour force, which is treated as synonymous with society at large. To define that class, use is made of either or both of two characteristics, both of which are measured by reference to official statistics.

The first characteristic – years of formal education required for employment in particular jobs – has been used both by those concerned with the professional 'class' in contemporary society (e.g. Ben-David, 1964; Bell, 1976) and those concerned with the role of professionals in complex productive organisations (e.g. Blau and Schoenherr, 1971). Essentially, they delineate professional workers as all those whose work is considered by employers to require four years of post-secondary education. In this sense, 'professionalisation' consists in the increase of the proportion of jobs in a society which require formal higher education. There can be little doubt that a trend of such an increase has existed in the past and that, for a variety of reasons, it will continue into the future. The same may be said for the second of the two common methods of delineating 'professions' as a stratum of the work force – that which singles out a group of workers who possess special knowledge (usually distinguished as abstract and theoretical) and skill (usually characterised as requiring the exercise of complex judgement). Patently, both formal education and skill or knowledge are closely related, for the latter may be said to have been inculcated by the former, and the former may be treated as a convenient institutional measure of the latter. In any case, the proportion of professionally skilled workers has been increasing in the labour force and is likely to continue to increase in the future. Thus, by educational and skill criteria, the professionalisation of the labour force will increase in the future.

The problem with both of these definitions of profession as a stratum of the labour force lies in their helpless dependence upon the governmental and managerial processes which create the categories both in official labour statistics and in managerial tables of organisation. Having no direct access to the workers or their work (and indeed, concerned less with the study of the institutions of productive work than with stratification as such), both definitions are in danger of dealing with official artefacts instead of the phenomena themselves. The requirement of formal education and the skill classification of workers may reflect institutional processes more than functional necessity. What is delineated by such definitions and measures of professions may not be the strictly functional necessities for the performance of a particular class of productive labour, so much as the institutional requirements for access to particular jobs, and institutional processes for classifying such jobs for reasons unrelated to the needs of productivity. Indeed, recent analysts such as Berg (1970) have argued that educational requirements for many jobs in the United States have been inflated beyond what is necessary for their adequate performance (cf. Collins, 1971: 1002-1019). And Braverman (1974: 426-435) has argued that skill-classifications of jobs have also been inflated well beyond the actual skill and judgement they require. Thus, while 'professionalisation' is, by measures of formal education and skill-classification, increasing, this increase may not reflect significant changes in the real education and skill required for effective productivity, may not reflect, in short, technological need for the 'centrality of theoretical knowledge' so important to the rationale of Bell's delineation of post-industrial society. The definition of 'profession' may thus refer more to how the powers that be in society or in productive organisations are prone to *classify* jobs than to the nature of the jobs themselves and the work experience of those who fill them.

A perhaps more serious deficiency in this usage of profession lies in the variety of occupations it includes, a variety of far-ranging and systematic differences so great that all those in the stratum cannot be seen to share anything more than higher education (no matter where or what substance) or a general skill-classification (no matter what the particular skill): nothing of any further significance is held in common. It is much too broad a classification to aid one to understand the differentiation of work and the processes of production (cf. Braverman, 1974: 403-409). The definition includes a large minority of the labour force, including both the traditional professionals and technicians. It in fact embraces what is designated as the 'professional and technical' ranks of labour in official classifications in the United States, and what is designated as the 'intelligentsia' in the Soviet Union (cf. Churchward, 1973). It includes much if not all of what some (cf. Mallet, 1975; Touraine, 1971) have called the 'new working class' and constitutes the growing segment of the labour force which Bell (1976: 15-18) sees as the major feature of the emergent society of the future.

Even a casual look at the array of occupations included in this broad 'professional' class reveals its analytical diffuseness. It includes physicians, engineers, dental technicians, clergymen, schoolteachers reporters, nurses, airline pilots, social workers, photographers, professors, chemists and a large and varied proportion labelled 'others'. So gross is the class that even Bell (1976: 213ff and 375) felt obliged to stratify it internally so as to separate an internal 'professional class' from 'semi-professions' and technicians. What joins all those occupations together into a single professional stratum is trivial compared to the nature of the differences between many of them. Neither general level of skill imputed by employers nor the amount of formal education required by employers tells us enough to allow us to analyse and explain the markedly different life-chances and work-lives of the occupations included in it. The problem with this usage of 'professional' thus lies in part in the empirically and theoretically problematic character of the criteria of formal education and imputed skill, but also no less importantly in the analytical limitations of class analysis itself. Class analysis is simply too gross to analyse the division of labour and the institutions of production in a society. To understand better the division of labour and the institutions of production, and to understand the crucial differences *among* occupations, I believe, requires instead an emphasis on the degree to which they, as occupations rather than classes, have gained the organised power to control themselves the terms, conditions and content of their work in the settings where they perform their work.

The Future of Occupational Monopoly and Dominance

A criterion of professionalisation other than skill or education is provided by a number of recent writings which all converge on the same emphasis. In work carried on in the tradition of occupational analysis (cf. Stewart and Cantor, 1974: 1-7), the attempt has been made to find strategic ways of distinguishing among occupations with almost equal education and skill but with markedly different working conditions – ways of distinguishing, for example, between pharmacists and optometrists in the contemporary United States (Freidson, 1970) – and ways of analysing markedly different situations for the 'same' occupation in different historical periods (Elliott, 1972: 14-57) and different national settings (Johnson, 1973: 281-309). What seemed critical in explaining those differences was the presence or absence of the organised power of the workers themselves to control the terms, conditions and content of their work – what Johnson (1972:45) called *collegiate control*, or 'professionalism'. Another way of delineating this approach is to be found in Weber's discussion of group monopoly (Weber, 1968: 339-348 and Berlant, 1975: 43-63).

The existence of such control over work by the workers themselves cannot be explained by the mere length or content of formal education or by some intrinsic character of skill. Rather, control presupposes a successful political organisation which can gain the power to negotiate and establish favourable jurisdictions in an organised division of labour, and to control the labour market. Variation in control may be seen as the critical difference between such occupations as pharmacist and physician. Both are nominal members of the 'professional class', both have complex skill, both have a higher education in the United States, and both have exclusive licences by which they monopolise certain tasks. But there is a critical difference between them: the pharmacist can work only at the order of the physician, and thus may be seen to be in a critically different position in the division of labour. It is possible to reserve the term 'profession' for that form of occupational organisation which has at once gained for its members a labour monopoly and a place in the division of labour that is free of the authority of others over their work. Work as such, and the skills it entails, while not irrelevant, are not the focus for discrimination so much as the organised place of an occupation in the labour market and in a division of labour. A particular kind of work – practice of the tasks of healing, for example – can be organised as a profession at one point in history and not at another, and in one nation and not another.

In assessing the analytical importance of occupational monopoly and authority as central criteria for differentiating labour, one must remember how pervasive can be its consequences. The recent position of medicine is a case in point (cf. Turner and Hodge, 1970: 38-41). The profession has been able to determine how many physicians are trained, who is selected to be trained, how they are to be trained, and who is to be licensed and thus to work. In that way it has controlled the labour market for its services. Furthermore, it has exercised supervisory power over a growing array of technical workers – the paraprofessional workers who may not work without authorisation or whose products (like laboratory analyses, X-rays) are unusable by anyone but physicians. In that way it has dominated a division of labour. Its control both restricts the supply of its own labour and subordinates related labour in the institutions in which its members work.

Most of medicine's control has not been exercised directly in negotiation with clients or employers, but rather indirectly, through licensing, registering and certifying legislation that establishes constraining limits around what can be negotiated among workers and with managers in concrete settings. As the Webbs noted some time ago (1917:

41), professional associations have found 'legal enactment even more advantageous in securing their own ends than the Trade Unions have hitherto done, and the organization and direction of political activity have become important features of the modern Professional Association'. Those organised powers of professional occupations have been real and are well known. Economists have deplored their interference with the labour market and thus, as labour monopolies, their purported cost to the public (Friedman, 1962); political scientists and lawyers have deplored their role as 'private governments' (Gilb, 1966; Lieberman, 1970).

Legislation is a more effective method of controlling the circumstances of work of the self-employed worker than is collective bargaining, but even employment of the worker does not in itself reduce the effective possibilties of occupational control. The effectively organised professional occupation controls even the determination and demarcation of tasks embodied in jobs supported by employers. There is no intrinsic reason why management in any particular organisation must be the agent, as it has been traditionally in industry, to determine what kind of worker must be hired for a particular job, what tasks those in and around that job can perform, and who can supervise and take responsibility for the proper performance of those jobs. Through their influence on regulatory agencies, the organised professions (and the crafts) are often responsible for writing the job descriptions for their members and determining the employer's training and educational requirements as well as the kind of special skill imputed to the qualified worker. They have done this independently of the employing organisation, and the employing organisation has been required by the state to follow those professionally determined guidelines in order to gain state charters or licences to operate. When an occupation gains effective organisation, therefore, it can raise powerful barriers against the process of rationalisation which management has been fairly free to advance in the case of those less-than-professionally organised technical workers who were recently discussed by Harries-Jenkins (1970: 53-107).

Given this definition of profession as an occupational monopoly with a position of dominance in a division of labour, what is the likelihood of professionalising more occupations in the future? What of the new technical occupations – those with more education and complex skill than most workers? By and large, Touraine seems accurate in describing them as largely powerless, and with few hopeful prospects (Touraine, 1971: 58). But this does not seem to be so because of the character of their higher education, knowledge or skill. Nor does it seem to have much to do with their salaried status. Rather, such occupations seem to have few prospects because they are part of productive domains which are already organised and controlled either (1) by dominant professions and their allies, or (2) by managerial agents of either the state (in socialist nations) or corporate capital. In the massive and still growing domains of health, welfare, law and education, the division of labour is organised around the central authority of dominant professions (Freidson, 1970: 47-84). In manufacturing, sales, financial, service and other such enterprises, the division of labour is organised by what Johnson referred to as 'corporate patronage' (Johnson, 1972: 46) – control by managerial authorities guided by elaborate information, plans and advice drawn up for them by a small corps of professionalised experts who constitute what Galbraith called the 'technostructure', and who are often mislabelled 'technocrats'.

In the former instance of professional dominance, the growing corps of technical workers is organised *around* the delineating and supervising authority of key professions. When they are licensed, certified or registered, the legitimacy, even the legality of their work hinges upon their nominal supervision by that dominant profession; in many cases, only the dominant profession can order, interpret, evaluate and consume the service they provide. They are thus bound into an occupationally subordinate position even though many have organised themselves into occupational associations and trade unions and have claimed many of the attributes ascribed to professions. Some of them may break away to occupy a niche in the division of labour that is parallel to and unsubordinated to their erstwhile occupational superiors, but most, in spite of their many 'professional' attributes, are certain to remain either, by my usage, paraprofessional workers, or to become transformed by managerial authority into technical workers with fewer of the trappings of professionalism. Trade unionism, I would guess, will succeed in improving the terms and conditions of their work, but will be unlikely to change their position as workers whose work is ultimately at the disposition of others (cf. Mann, 1973: 20-21).

In those industries where there is managerial dominance, the technician is also unlikely to gain control over his work because, apart from the general training he brings with him into his job, his work tends to be a function of the needs of a particular job defined by a particular organisation. This specificity of task, over which he has little control, prevents his actual working skills from being generalisable across a wide variety of jobs, thereby hampering both individual job mobility and the possibility of developing collegial solidarity across employing organisations (Mallet, 1975: 68-75, saw 'sectoralism' or *internal* solidarity as a possible outcome). Furthermore, unorganised to begin with, he is likely to be able to wield little power to prevent periodic managerial rationalisation and the adoption of new techniques which threaten him with the spectre of his own obsolescence, or replacement by a machine. Under those circumstances, his development of organised control over his own work is unlikely. Indeed, as Goldner and Ritti (1967: 489-502) noted for the engineer, technician *par excellence,* 'professionalisation' may constitute in reality only a flattering symbolic reward by management to conceal career immobility and even demotion in those circumstances in which true career success is gained by leaving one's occupation to join the ranks of management.

Finally, there is the matter of the future of the present-day occupations which now have extensive control over the terms, conditions and content of their work. This may not be a question we can answer by simple linear projection because different professions provide services to clientele who are constituted in significantly different ways, and perform tasks with markedly different implications for institutional control. Perhaps more important is a fairly recent threat to professions created by rising expectations for greater productivity – that is, for the wider distribution of more professionally produced goods and services through the population. This has led to the generation of political forces which are pressing toward important changes in the organisation and delineation of the work of present-day professions. While some decline in relative prestige and income is entirely possible in the future, and while *portions* of presently professional work may very well return to the control of lay persons or become controlled by management, none of those changes has any intrinsic or inevitable connection with loss of occupational monopoly or position in the division of labour and most writers do not anticipate such a loss in the future. Very recently, however, a few writers (e.g. Haug, 1973, Haug, 1975, Oppenheimer, 1973) have pointed to trends which they employ as evidence that the future will bring changes in status so extreme as to lead to either deprofessionalisation or proletarianisation. Much of their argument is empirically unverifiable, and as is characteristic of the literature in general, it is not entirely certain that they are all talking about the same occupations, but some of their argument is based on three long-standing trends which are unquestionable, and which therefore deserve close attention. Let us examine those trends and their implications for assessing the future of professionalisation.

First, the trend toward specialisation *within* the established professions – a trend almost certain to continue – is argued to be contributory to deprofessionalisation or proletarianisation in that increasingly narrow specialists can be expected, like the classic factory worker, to be doing the same work over and over again, without knowledge or control of the whole productive process of which each specialty is a mere part. True as far as it goes, such reasoning is based on confusing two profoundly different processes of developing and organising specialisation. In one, very common in the history of crafts and professions, *the workers themselves* specialise and negotiate with their fellow workers for a niche *within* the occupation's division of labour. They do not lose organised control over their work. In the other, characteristic of the experience of the factory worker, *a superior authority* breaks a task down into its simplest units, requiring the least possible skill to perform, and then hires, trains and supervises workers to perform them in a division of labour it creates. In both instances specialisation does indeed occur, but in the former case it is the worker who invents, chooses and controls his task, trains for it in depth and pursues its minutest complexity on the basis of increasingly esoteric skill, while in the latter case it is management that creates a task which has been broken into specialised activities requiring little training or skill and the use of workers who are cheap and readily interchangeable (cf. Braverman, 1974: 85-121). Both are indeed 'specialisation', but an increase in the development of the former within the professions cannot be said to be analogous to the development of the latter, which dissolves traditional occupational jurisdictions. Evidence of managerial creation and control of work would have to be demonstrated before claims of deprofessionalisation or proletarianisation could be supported. No such evidence has been produced. The bald fact of an increase in specialisation without reference to evidence about the way it is developed and organised thus has little analytical relevance to the issue.

Second, the trend toward increasing complexity in the division of labour of which professionals are merely one part has been adduced to sustain the prophecy of deprofessionalisation or proletarianisation. The trend toward a more elaborate division of labour is as indubitable as that toward specialisation *within* professions, and represents part of the same process, but it, too, means little when treated as a mere quantitative phenomenon. Specialisation and the division of labour have indeterminate analytical significance without consideration of their social organisation (Freidson, 1976b). It is true that when one who once worked by himself comes to work as part of a larger division of labour, he becomes one interdependent part of a larger whole, but as the political theory of centuries has observed, interdependence does not mean each part of the whole has equal authority. In present-day health care, a professionalised industry in which the division of labour has grown increasingly complex for fifty years or more, there is little or no evidence that physicians have been losing significant elements of their monopoly over ordering and supervising the work provided by other occupations in the division of labour. Interdependence does not necessarily corrode dominance. The empirical examples of exceptions to professional dominance cited to support prophecies of the deprofessionalisation or proletarianisation of physicians are drawn from special experimental programmes in artificial (usually academic) settings, or from temporary arrangements observed in times of institutional or national crisis. Provocative and worth study as they may be, such exceptions are cross-sectional in nature and do *not* constitute trend data on which sound prophecy can be based.

Finally, there is the long-remarked (cf. Marshall, 1939; Lewis and Maude, 1952) trend away from self-employment and towards employment in large organisations. As an indicator this also is much too mechanical to have analytical value in and of itself. For one thing, priests, rabbis and ministers in organised churches have almost never been self-employed. The same may be said for the university teacher, at least since the demise of the mediaeval university, and for the modern research scientist. Does this mean that all this time they have really been members of the proletariat? Employment does indeed indicate nominal dependence on another agent to provide one's income, but so also does self-employment. The analytical issue is not employment or self-employment as such so much as the nature of the process by which the content, terms and conditions of work are established. If workers have a monopoly in the labour market, and the power to control their own work, they can dictate the content, terms and conditions of their employment as well as of their self-employment. Without monopoly and dominance their position when self-employed is hardly less desperate than when employed, as anyone familiar with the history of medical and legal self-employment should be aware. Furthermore, presently available large-scale data on employment and self-employment – particularly in the case of traditionally self-employed professions – is unreliable because of the artifactual character of the designations. Of the increasing proportion of American physicians who are now classified as employees, a significant number are shareowners of an incorporated practice organisation who are on a salary solely for legal and tax convenience. This does not imply that they have become a proletariat any more than does the fact that workers in worker-managed enterprises are usually paid wages. The fact of being employed or self-employed, then, is too ambiguous a datum to serve as useful evidence bearing on the future of professional monopoly and dominance.

What, then, can we say of the future of professional monopoly and dominance in a division of labour? First, it seems difficult to see any trend by which many more occupations will move into such a professional position (cf. Wilensky, 1963: 137-158). The trend in industrial societies has indeed been toward more licensing, registration and certification of occupations, providing them with a monopoly in the labour market, but there does not seem to be a trend toward occupations assuming new positions of over-all dominance in a division of labour. Second, it seems difficult to see any trend toward significant expansion in both numbers and functions of present-day established professions that does not at the same time imply radical changes in their constitution. The trend instead seems to be toward a redefinition of both function and jurisdiction. In all industrial countries, the cost of the comparatively long period of training now given professionals has become too great to allow them and only them to meet individual and public demand for all the services they now monopolise. This would be so even were their compensation to be reduced to a considerably more modest level than at present. Sooner or later, many of the more common and putatively less complex skills now monopolised by professionals will be transferred into the hands of less expesively trained workers who will be allowed some form of limited practice. This could take place both by the use of non-professionals, and by the sharpening and deepening of the stratification presently existing in the professions, with the lower stratum, increased in size, receiving shortened training and considerably more restricted rights to practise.

If the reorganisation of jurisdiction and task occurs, the essential analytical issue for the future of professions lies in the way in which this will come about, who will guide the process and specify the options and who will control it. Judging by the experience of state socialist nations which have attempted drastic changes in the political and legal status of the established professions, political ideology and power can effectively enforce the choice of broad goals and means available to professionalised work, but the professions have remained in control of the knowledge and technique by which those goals and the broad means connected with them are advanced. It seems unlikely that in the course of reorganisation there will be a reproduction of the process that occurred in manufacturing, with present-day professional workers losing control of the knowledge and technique connected with their work. Even if the number of their members falls and their present-day tasks are taken over by non-professionals, there is likely to remain in the future an important place for the professions, at the very least as planners and programmers of the reorganisation of their erstwhile work, as researchers and teachers, and as consultants to and supervisors of the workers who have replaced them in the provision of direct services.

The Future of Committed Labour

Thus far, my discussion has been limited to positional and structural characteristics which deal with relations to the market, strata within the entire labour force, and occupational organisation as it is manifested in a labour market and a division of labour. These modes of analysis all lack reference to human beings, and to the commitments, relationships and values that are, at bottom, what they purport to analyse. In addition to this analytical deficiency, one may note the absence, thus far, of any reference to one of the most commonly cited characteristics employed to define professions – the orientation to ethical service of others. Many scholars have emphasised such dedication: to cite just a few examples, Goode (1960: 903) has stressed as one of two 'core characteristics' of professions an orientation to serving the public good. Halmos (1970) claimed altruism. Tawney (1920: 94) and Carr-Saunders and Wilson (1933: 284-286) emphasised the significance of the professional's sense of responsibility for the integrity of his work. In general, such discussions do not refer to the social organisation of professional work so much as to the motivations and values of professional workers.

Elsewhere (Freidson, 1970: 77-82) I have discussed the problem of determining the empirical referents of such imputed attributes of professional workers, and I have questioned their validity as empirical statements about professionals. Whether or not the substance of those attributes is empirically accurate, however, the *class* of variable they represent is essential to address in any systematic analysis of work and workers, for values and motivation cannot be ignored. The problem with traditional discussions of 'ethicality' lies not in the unimportance of the topic, but in their level of abstraction and in their tendency to treat the topic as if it were something to be merely added to a list of other attributes, without relating each to each. While this is not the place for a detailed exposition, and while I do not claim that it is the only useful method of relating traditional attributes to each other, I wish to suggest here that the social psychology of professions and professionals can be discussed coherently and systematically as derivations from the social organisation of professions.

In essence, it can be argued that the social organisation of professions constitutes circumstances which encourage the development in its members of several kinds of commitment. (On commitment, see Becker, 1970: 261-273.) First, since an organised occupation provides its members with the prospect of a relatively secure and life-long career, it is reasonable to expect them to develop a commitment to and identification with the occupation and its fortunes, if only on self-interested, economic grounds. Such *occupational commitment* is markedly different from what is found in prototypical wage labour, whose commitment is not to a particular *occupation* but only to whatever job provides the most material benefit. Second, since an organised occupation by definition controls recruitment, training and job characteristics, its members will have many more common occupational experiences in training, job career and work than is the case for members of a general skill class, who are recruited, trained and employed in a considerably more heterogeneous fashion in the course of their work lives. Such shared experience – sometimes referred to as occupational culture or occupational community (Salaman, 1974) – in conjunction with sharing the occupation's privileged (and sometimes threatened) position in the labour market and the division of labour, may be seen to encourage commitment to colleagues, or collegiality. Such *occupational solidarity* tends to be exclusive in character, rather than extending across occupations to a working class. Third, we may see professional organisation encouraging *work commitment*. In so far as jurisdictional boundaries are comparatively stable, they allow the performance of a set of particular tasks for a lifetime. This provides the opportunity and stimulus for the worker to develop a committed interest in the work he performs. Work can become a central life interest for professionals far more easily than for blue-collar workers (cf. Dubin, 1956: 131-142 and Orzack, 1959: 125-132), for the latter cannot be assured of performing the same tasks from one job to the next, let alone perform tasks that they create and control themselves.

Occupational organisation may thus be related to workers' commitment to and identification with their occupation, their occupational coworkers, and their work. But what does this have to do with dedication, altruism, service orientation or craftsmanship? (On craftsmanship, see Mills, 1951: 220-224.) Can they, too, be said to have some plausible connection with occupational organisation? When this is discussed in the literature, the consensus seems to be – paralleling the claims of the professions themselves – that professions recruit members who are devoted to serving others, create training programmes which instill dedication to serve others, and organise work settings in such a way that altruistic and craftsmanlike work is assured by informal processes of collegial control. That is to say, the theory is that the content of the institutions sustained by professional organisation is such as to encourage and maintain dedication in members.

Dedication implies that what is unique to professions is not the fact of having a material relationship to a market – as in the case of the professional/amateur distinction discussed earlier in this paper – but rather the fact of being a literal amateur – of working for the love of others and for the love of the work rather than for the love of money. But in the world as we find it, market relations and the social organisation of the means of production are more apparent to the observer than is dedication. Empirical evidence does not support the claim of a distinctive dedication which takes precedence over individual and collective material interest. In a recently reported study of a group of doctors (Freidson, 1976a), it was shown how etiquette – an expression of occupational solidarity – was given priority over efforts to realise the ideals of dedication to service and to craftsmanship. Without denying that on some occasions and in some individuals those ideals are empirically realised, there is little evidence that they are distinctive for professionals or correlated with professional organisation. Indeed, I would suggest that the notions of dedication to service and of craftsmanship are more usefully treated as elements of an ideology than as empirical characteristics of individual and collective professional behaviour. Taken as ideology, they have empirical status as claims about their members made by occupations attempting to gain and maintain professional monopoly and dominance.

Certainly it is evident that ideologies of craftsmanship and public service are advanced by workers attempting to gain and maintain control over the determination of their own work and working conditions (cf. Jamous and Peloille, 1970: 111-152 and Holzner, 1972). Since such control hinges on gaining access to power which is not inherent in the work itself, an ideology of professionalism must be ecumenical rather than parochial (cf. Dibble, 1962), designed to persuade those in power that members of the occupation are the best arbiters of the work, that the work is in the public interest, and that the workers are dedicated to doing good work and using their privilege for the good of others rather than for their own interests alone. That ideology may be said to be an important component of the process by which occupations seek to gain and maintain their control.

There is, however, more use for the ideology of professionalism than just the advancement of the ends of workers in an organised occupation. It may also be used to motivate workers in the *absence* of occupational control over work. Involvement in and commitment to work, and an orientation toward service, have been found among non-professional workers whose occupational position prevents them from controlling their own work. Indeed, those working under the direction of professionals may very well manifest greater devotion to serving others than do professionals themselves (see, e.g. Hall, 1968: 97 and Engel, 1973). Organisational superiors can use the ideology to make career immobility and even demotion palatable to workers (Goldner and Ritti, 1967), as can professionals in the course of passing down 'dirty work' to subordinate occupations (Emerson and Pollner, 1976: 243-254). The ideology is not only attached to the armamentarium of professional occupations, therefore, but also employed by occupation leaders aspiring to professional status, by members of occupations subordinate to professions, and by members of occupations like engineering which have an uncertain status in a managerially dominated system. The ideology may be used by political, managerial and professional authorities to distract workers from their objective lack of control over their work, to lead them to do the work assigned them as well as possible, and to commit them to means and ends others have chosen for them.

In sum, it is possible to observe that occupational commitment may be plausibly treated as a function of professional organisation, varying directly in strength and frequency as occupational organisation varies. The same may be said for work commitment. So also may it be said for occupational solidarity, though the strength of the association may be diminished by internal differentiation into specialties and segments within a profession. The futures of each of these commitments may thus be expected to be tied up intimately with the future of occupational monopoly and dominance. Commitment to serving others, however, and to doing good work, cannot be connected so plausibly with occupational organisation, and remains analytically separate from it except as an ideology that aids its development and maintenance. Espousal of the ideology by individuals may be empirically present even when the professional organisation of work is absent, for it does not seem to depend upon professional monopoly and control for its existence. Thus, even though professional organisation should decline in the future, the use of the ideology of professionalism could very well increase.

The Futures of Professionalisation

I began this paper by noting that a large number of eminent writers over many decades have seen a trend toward the increase of professions in the future. I expressed doubt that they all agreed with each other on much more than the use of the same word, and suggested that they may in fact be talking past each other even when they appeared to agree, let alone when they disagreed. I suggested a careful look at the varied referents of the word, and in the body of my paper did so, examining the varied referents both for their analytical value and for assessing the trends in their development in the future.

With my discussion of profession as an ideology, as a claim of dedication advanced to protect an interest, I came to the end of the catalogue. I have not been exhaustive of all the attributes which have composed all the definitions of the term, but I believe I have touched on the most essential. Even if I have overlooked some of importance, I trust I have made the point that what one predicts as the future of professions is based on one's conception of what they are, in interaction with the evidence of trends. For a term like 'profession', used in so many ways, there cannot be sufficient consensus in usage and definition to make it possible to predict only one future. There can only be many futures, each a function of choice of definition and each correct within the limits of the available data and its own definition.

One might observe furthermore that two different predictions can be at the same time accurate in the light of available data and completely contradictory of each other. This can be so because the criteria or attributes employed in one prediction may have no relationship to those employed in the other, so that each can use data that vary independently of the other. Thus, defining professions as occupations with higher education and imputed complex skill yields a prediction of continuing increase in the future; defining professions as self-employed occupations yields a prediction of continuing decrease in the future; defining professions by monopoly and dominance in a division of labour yields a prediction of at best slight increase and possible mild decrease. Definitions may also be related to some but not all others: taken as dependent variable, commitment to occupation, fellow workers and work may be seen to vary with occupational organisation, but it is likely to vary slightly with, and perhaps even independently of education and imputed skill. Dedication to service and to craftsmanship, on the other hand, may be seen to have no simple and direct relationship to any of the other criteria of professionalisation discussed here: as ideologies, they seem to be available for the use of any agent seeking to control work and motivate and direct the worker.

Finally, I might note that in this paper there is another perhaps more important theme running alongside the issue of defining and predicting professionalisation. It argues that a fruitful way of developing theoretical coherence in the field of the sociology of occupations lies in adopting as one's central problem the analysis of the organisation of control over work, and its consequences for work, workers, organisations and society. Part of the virtue of such a focus lies in its compatability with other bodies of information and theory which have heretofore run largely separate from occupational sociology as a discipline. When individual occupations are seen as part of a division of labour composed of many occupations, much of organisational theory becomes relevant as an explication of particular ways of organising and coordinating an institutional division of labour. So, also, does much of the work in industrial sociology. This focus, then, can join occupational sociology to other specialties, and advance intellectual synthesis. Perhaps more important, on the level of general theory, focus on the issue of control over work facilitates the critical use of at least some of the perspectives and analytical tools developed by Marxist theory, which contains at its core the same emphasis on control even though its preoccupation is more with analysis of class than of occupation. But that is all programmatic: what is important here is the exploration of the analytical meaning of the various attributes employed to delineate professions, and the direction it points toward future analysis of an important, even though ambiguous phenomenon of industrial society.

Notes

1. Revision of a Plenary address at the Annual Conference of the British Sociological Association, Manchester, England, 9 April 1976. This paper is based on work partially supported by the Russell Sage Foundation. It has benefited from critical comments and suggestions by Howard S. Becker, Arlene K. Daniels, Celia Davies, William A. Form, Richard H. Hall, Marie R. Haug, Carol L. Kronus, John B. McKinlay, Caroline Persell, Margaret E. Reid and Dennis H. Wrong.
2. It will be recognised as Max Weber's definition of *Beruf*, which the translator interprets as 'occupation'. (See Weber, 1947: 250.)
3. It is true that on official forms it is proper to list 'housewife', 'student' and 'retired' as one's 'occupation', but that practice is more a matter of denying

the stigma of unemployment than of claiming an official position in the labour force.

References

Becker, Howard S. (1970). *Sociological Work.* Chicago, Aldine Publishing Co.

Bell, Daniel. (1976). *The Coming of Post-Industrial Society.* New York, Basic Books.

Ben-David, Joseph. (1964). 'Professions in the class system of present-day societies', *Current Sociology,* vol. 12, pp. 247-330.

Berg, Ivar. (1970). *Education and Jobs: The Great Training Robbery.* New York, Praeger Publishers.

Berlant, Jeffrey Lionel. (1975). *Profession and Monopoly.* Berkeley, University of California Press.

Blau, Peter and Richard A. Schoenherr. (1971). *The Structure of Organizations.* New York, Basic Books.

Carr-Saunders, A.M. (1928). *Professions: Their Organization and Place in Society.* Oxford, The Clarendon Press.

Carr-Saunders, A.M. and P.A. Wilson. (1933). *The Professions.* Oxford, Clarendon Press.

Churchward, L.G. (1973). *The Soviet Intelligentsia. An Essay on the Social Structure and Roles of the Soviet Intellectuals.* Boston, Routledge and Kegan Paul.

Collins, Randall. (1971). 'Functional and conflict theories of educational stratification', *American Sociological Review,* vol. 36, December, pp. 1002-19.

Dibble, Vernon K. (1962). 'Occupations and ideologies', *American Journal of Sociology,* vol. 68, September, pp. 229-41.

Dubin, Robert. (1956). 'Industrial workers' worlds: a study of the 'central life interests' of industrial workers', *Social Problems,* vol. 3, January, pp. 131-42.

Elliott, Philip. (1972). *The Sociology of the Professions.* London, Macmillan.

Emerson, Robert M. and Melvin Pollner. (1976). 'Dirty work designations: their features and consequences in a psychiatric setting', *Social Problems,* vol. 23, February, pp. 243-54.

Engel, Gloria V. (1973). 'Social factors affecting the work satisfaction of the physician's assistant', *Sociological Review Monograph,* no. 20, pp. 245-61.

Freidson, Eliot. (1970). *Profession of Medicine: A Study in the Sociology of Applied Knowledge.* New York, Dodd, Mead.

— (1976a). *Doctoring Together: A Study of Professional Social Control.* New York, Elsevier Publishing Co.

— 1976b. 'The division of labor as social interaction', *Social Problems,* vol. 23, February, pp. 304-13.

Friedman, Milton. (1962). *Capitalism and Freedom.* Chicago, University of Chicago Press.

Gilb, Corrine L. (1966). *Hidden Hierarchies: The Professions and Government.* New York, Harper and Row.

Goldner, Fred and R.R. Ritti. (1967). 'Professionalism as career immobility', *American Journal of Sociology,* vol. 72, March, pp. 489-502.

Goode, William J. (1960). 'Encroachment, charlatanism, and the emerging profession: psychology, medicine and sociology', *American Sociological Review,* vol. 25, pp. 902-14.

Habenstein, Robert. (1963). 'Critique of "profession" as a sociological category', *Sociological Quarterly,* vol. 4, Autumn, pp. 291-300.

Hall, Richard H. (1968). 'Professionalization and bureaucratization', *American Sociological Review,* vol. 33, February, p. 97.

—(1975). *Occupations and the Social Structure,* 2nd ed. Englewood Cliffs, N.J. Prentice-Hall.
Halmos, Paul. (1970). *The Personal Service Society.* New York, Schocken Books.
Harries-Jenkins, G. (1970). 'Professionals in organizations', in J.A. Jackson (ed.), *Professions and Professionalization.* Cambridge, Cambridge University Press, pp. 53-107.
Haug, Marie R. (1973). 'Deprofessionalization: an alternative hypothesis for the future', *Sociological Review Monograph,* no. 20, pp. 195-211.
— (1975). 'The deprofessionalization of everyone?', *Sociological Focus,* vol. 8, August, pp. 197-213.
Holzner, Burkart. (1972). *Reality Construction in Society.* Cambridge, Mass., Schenkman Publishing Co.
Horn, Joshua S. (1969). *Away With all Pests.* New York, Monthly Review Press.
Hughes, Everett C. (1971). *The Sociological Eye.* Chicago, Aldine Publishing Co.
Jaffe, Abraham J. (1968). Labor force: definitions and measurement. *International Encyclopedia of the Social Sciences.* vol. 8. New York, Macmillan and The Free Press, pp. 469-74.
Jamous, H. and B. Peloille. (1970). 'Changes in the French university hospital system'. In J.A. Jackson (ed.), *Professions and Professionalization.* Cambridge, Cambridge University Press, pp. 11-152.
Johnson, Terence J. (1972). *Professions and Power.* London, Macmillan.
— (1973). Imperialism and the professions', *Sociological Review Monograph,* no. 20, pp. 281-309.
Lewis, Roy and Angus Maude. (1952). *Professional People.* London. Phoenix House.
Lieberman, Jethro K. (1970). *The Tyranny of the Experts.* New York, Walker and Co.
Mann, Michael. (1973). *Consciousness and Action among the Western Working Class.* London, Macmillan.
Mallet, Serge. (1975). *The New Working Class.* Nottingham, Spokeman Books.
Marshall, T.H. (1939). 'The recent history of professionalism in relation to social structure and social policy', *Canadian Journal of Economics and Political Science,* vol. 5 August, pp. 325-40.
Millerson, Geoffrey. (1964). *The Qualifying Associations: A Study in Professionalization.* London, Routledge and Kegan Paul.
Mills, C. Wright. (1951). *White Collar.* New York, Oxford University Press.
Mincer, Jacob. (1968). 'Labor force: participation', *International Encyclopedia of the Social Sciences.* vol. 8. New York, Macmillan and Free Press, pp. 474-81.
Oakley, Ann. (1974). *The Sociology of Housework.* New York, Pantheon Books.
Oppenheimer, Martin. (1973). 'The proletarianization of the professional', *Sociological Review Monograph*, no. 20, pp. 213-27.
Orzack, Louis H. (1959). 'Work as a "central life interest" of professionals', *Social Problems*, vol. 7, Fall, pp. 125-32.
Parsons, Talcott. (1968). 'Professions'. *International Encyclopedia of the Social Sciences.* vol. 12. New York, Macmillan and The Free Press, pp. 536-47.
Salaman, Graeme. (1974). *Community and Occupation.* Cambridge, Cambridge University Press.
Spencer, Herbert. (1896). *The Principles of Sociology.* New York, Appleton.
Stewart, Phyllis L. and Muriel G. Cantor. (1974). *Varieties of Work Experience.* Cambridge, Mass., Schenkman Publishing Co.
Tawney, R.H. (1920). *The Acquisitive Society.* New York, Harcourt Brace.
Touraine, Alain. (1971). *The Post-Industrial Society.* New York, Random House,
Turner, C. and M.N. Hodge. (1970). 'Occupations and professions'. In J.A. Jackson (ed.), *Professions and Professionalization.* Cambridge, Cambridge

University Press, pp. 38-41.
Webb, Sidney and Beatrice Webb. (1917). 'Special supplement on professional associations', *New Statesman,* 9 (no. 211, Saturday, 21 April).
Weber, Max. (1947). *The Theory of Social and Economic Organization.* New York, Oxford University Press.
— (1968). *Economy and Society.* vol. 1. New York, Bedminster Press.
Wilensky, Harold L. (1964). 'The professionalization of everyone?', *American Journal of Sociology,* vol. 70, September, pp. 137-58.

One of the commonest unacknowledged biases of much contemporary sociology derives from its leading practitioners' social and institutional bases in urban areas in advanced liberal democracies. Most work in the medical profession and other health care occupations derives, implicitly or explicitly, from experience in North America or Northern Europe. Jesús de Miguel's discussion of Spain is therefore welcome for the information which it offers on a country whose social organisation remains mysterious.

In addition important lessons may be drawn from his survey. First, he underlines the need to take account of the political context of professional work. In Spain, despite the prestige accorded to doctors, their political influence is negligible, other than as members of a substantial urban bourgeoisie. Under an authoritarian régime, it is the political leadership which formulates and enforces policies to which doctors are, for the most part, willing accomplices. Unlike Britain or the USA, the medical profession has no substantial organisation free to act in opposition to the national political leadership in pressing for policies contrary to those favoured by the régime. De Miguel's comparison of Spain with Portugal emphasises that in Spain the co-option of the profession depend upon their membership of an affluent bourgeoisie, while in Portugal the medical profession tended to oppose the Salazar régime with little success.

Second, de Miguel's comments on the regional inequalities in health care provision are valuable. He shows how the alliance between the medical profession and a centralised authoritarian state has led to a concentration of doctors and other medical services in the richest parts of the richest cities of the richest regions. The doctors, and consequently most health care provision, have gravitated towards the affluent urban bourgeoisie which provide their social base. Clearly a non-democratic state could direct labour, if it had the will. But such a will would only arise if the political leadership drew its bases from rural or deprived urban areas, as in China or Cuba. The issue of centre-periphery relations within the UK has been much neglected by British sociologists, although problems associated with contemporary attempts to equalise the regional health care budgets show its importance. Under what conditions did centralisation develop in Britain and to what do we owe the present devolutionary pressures? De Miguel's analysis offers us one possible model and remedy in his advocacy of local and regional democracy as a way of relating health care provision to the needs of those whom it serves.

On the whole, though, de Miguel's paper is welcome as much for the data which it offers as for its substantive arguments.

R.D.

The editors would like to acknowledge the helpful comments of Dr Adrian Griffiths, London School of Hygiene and Tropical Medicine, in their editorial work, although responsibility for this version remains with Dr de Miguel and themselves.

THE ROLE OF THE MEDICAL PROFESSION IN A NON-DEMOCRATIC COUNTRY: THE CASE OF SPAIN

Jesús M. de Miguel*

This paper examines the structure, ideology, and conflicts of the medical profession in a non-democratic country, Spain. It is divided into three parts: (1) an overview of the structural peculiarities of the Spanish medical profession compared with other southern European countries (Portugal, Italy, Yugoslavia); (2) an analysis of the distinctive ideologies that Spanish physicians have developed during the years 1939 to 1976; and (3) a brief reference to the power conflicts between the medical profession and other pressure groups, as well as within the medical profession itself. This triple analysis attempts to contribute further research on the role of the medical profession in non-democratic countries to augment the models biased towards Western democracies which sociologists in this field have developed. It seeks to examine two different questions: (1) in what manner is the health structure[1] of a non-democratic country influenced by the manifest and latent objectives of the medical profession; and (2) in what ways is a social group, like the medical profession, shaped by the structure of a non-democratic society?

The Structure of the Medical Profession

The medical profession has been characterised by reference to features like autonomy, monopoly, organisation, action orientation, abstract knowledge, service orientation, status, charisma and the like.[2] However, all of these notions have different meanings in the context of democratic and non-democratic countries. Where the medical profession

*These pages are part of a paper presented at the British Sociological Association, 1976 Annual Conference (Manchester, 6-9 April 1976). Dr. Jesús M. de Miguel, Ph.D., is *profesor adjunto* in the Department of Sociology, Universitat Autonòma de Barcelona (Bellaterra, Barcelona, Spain). The author is deeply grateful to the critical aid of Melissa G. Moyer, the technical help of Mercedes González-Page, and the excellent editorial comments of Margaret Stacey. The research was indirectly supported by grants from the Social Science Research Council (New York), and the British Council. I also thank Mr Harold Normington for his interest and consideration. This study is part of an investigation on health manpower in Spain, directed by the author, of which a book has been published: *La reforma sanitaria en Espana* (Madrid: Cambio 16, 1977). A follow up of these ideas appears in J.M. de Miguel (ed.), *Planificación y reforma sanitarias* (Madrid: IOP, 1977).

enjoys high status, as in most Western countries, it tends to resist intrusion by other social groups and to reserve its monopoly for a limited number of members. Entrance into the profession is a long, costly and difficult process. In a non-democratic country the medical profession systematically uses its power to contain the growth in numbers of new physicians. This policy is more effective in capitalist countries than in socialist ones, where the status of the medical profession is generally lower. In Figure 1 we can observe the changes in the number of physicians in Europe between 1950 and 1970. The highest rate of growth is in the socialist countries, particularly Poland and Yugoslavia, although it must be remembered that these have very low initial bases; Romania follows more a Mediterranean than a socialist pattern; the Soviet Union has the highest ratio of physicians to population in the world (after Israel) but its growth is slow compared to other socialist countries possibly because it has a larger base in this period. Interestingly, the pattern for the next decade is that countries with a relatively high ratio of physicians to population will increase that ratio more rapidly than less developed countries. In the whole world, 'the differential mechanisms of population growth bring about the paradoxical situation in which the regions best supplied with physicians are also those which will have to exert the least effort in order to maintain the present level of medical density'.[3] As we can observe, Spain shows one of the lowest European rates of increase in the expansion of its medical profession partly because its doctor/population ratio was already relatively high, and partly because of the success of the established medical profession in keeping the number of physicians down.[4] In total there are about 50,000 physicians in Spain (1.4 per 1,000 inhabitants), 17,000 pharmacists and 7,000 veterinarians.

The increase in the numbers of physicians has not produced a better distribution. On the contrary, the regional differences have progressively widened. In Map 1 we observe the regional distribution of physicians (per 10,000 population) in four countries. Portugal presents the dramatic situation of a high concentration of physicians in Lisbon, Oporto and Coimbra, with the rest of the country unattended. Spain has a low rate of physicians in the south (except for the provinces with medical schools), and in Galicia in the northwest. In Italy, the central region (from Liguria and Emilia Romagna to Latium) has the highest rates of doctors while the *Mezzogiorno* has low rates. Finally, in Yugoslavia, we observe the patterns of a developed north (Slovenia), and a very retarded south (Kosovo-Metohia). However, the maldistribution of physicians in these countries is not the only regional problem.

Figure 1 Physicians in Europe 1950–1970

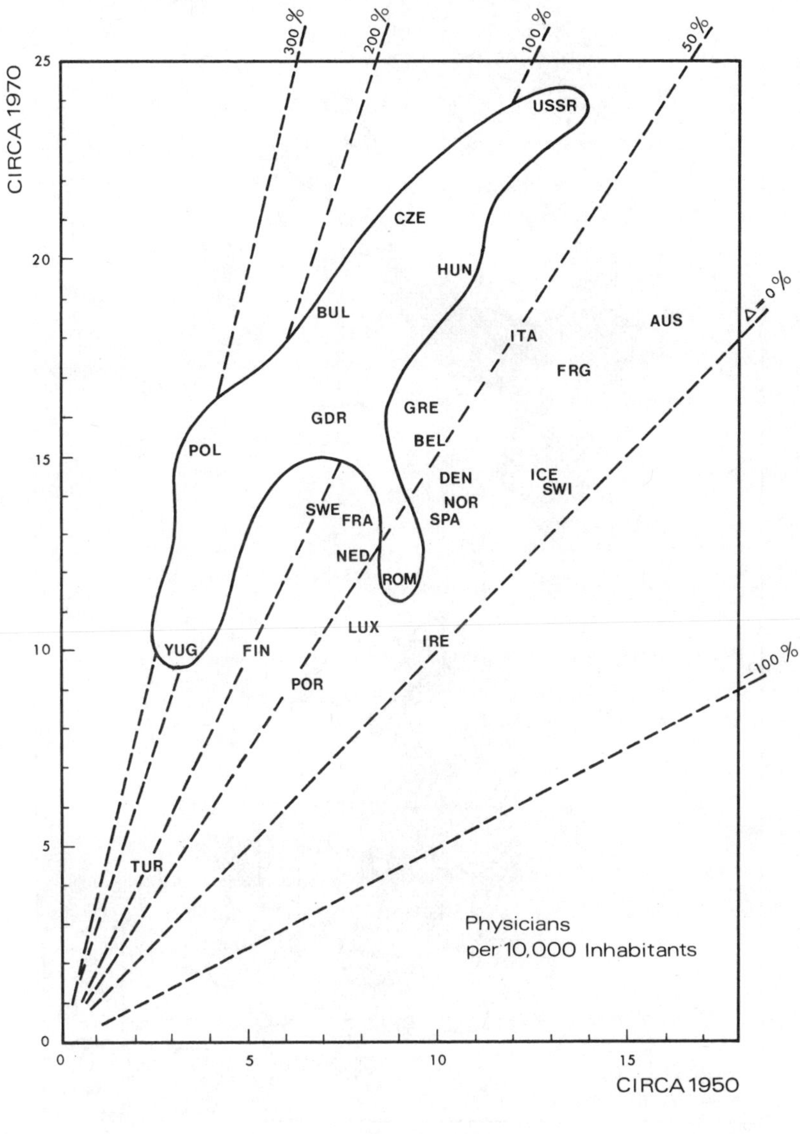

Source: WHO, *World Health Statistics Annual 1970.* vol. 3. pp. 120-22.

Map 1 Rate of Physicians in the Northern Mediterranean Region, circa 1972 (per 10,000 population)

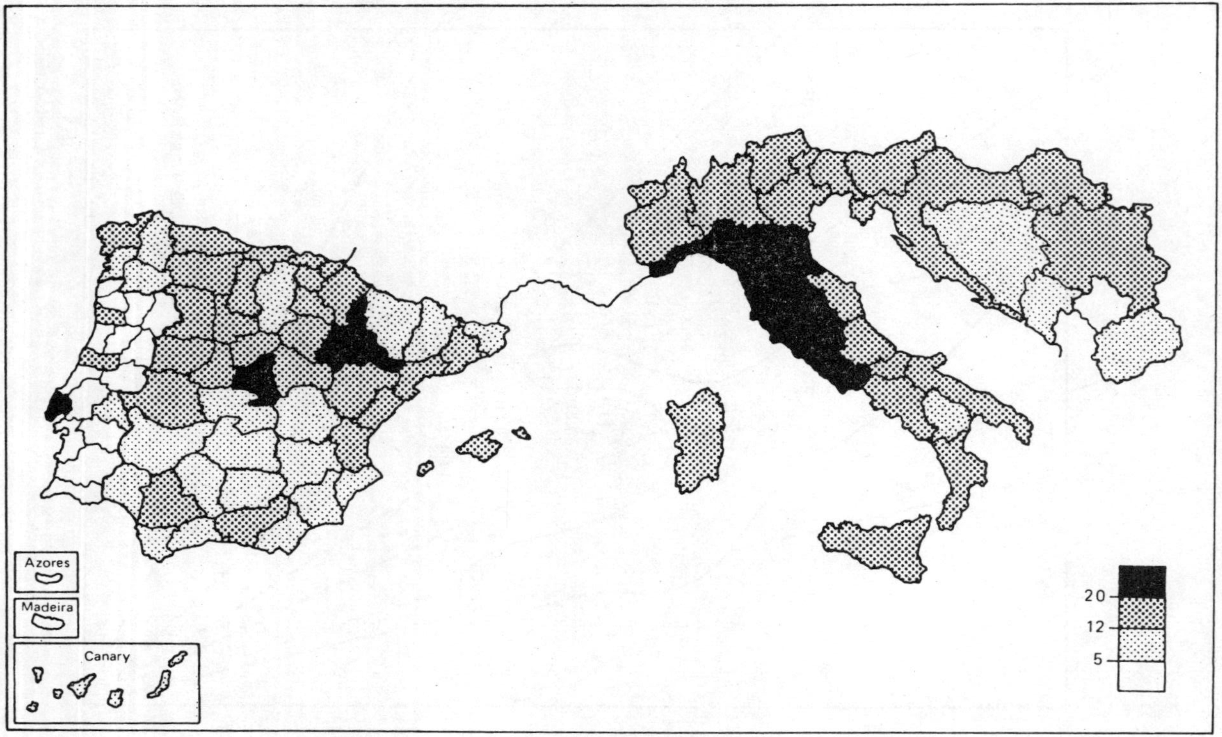

Differences by activities and specialisation are also found. From a regional point of view hospitals are even more inequitably distributed than physicians.

In the case of Spain the general pattern is to have higher rates of physicians in regions with higher levels of development, although several exceptions can be found. The provinces with medical schools present exceptionally high rates independently of their economic growth. At similar levels of development, Castile has higher rates than Andalusia or Galicia. If we observe the trend of the doctor/population ratio according to the level of economic development (measured by the percentage of active agrarian population) in 1960 and 1970, we may see how the slope of the trend is greatest for Madrid and Barcelona. Physicians are concentrated not only for reasons of economic development but also for administrative (or regional) centralism. The concentration of physicians is not only in the most developed regions but most of all in the cities of these regions. The two patterns are common to all countries in the world, but much more pronounced in those non-democratic countries where control over the medical profession by the population is minimal. For example, the six largest cities in Spain all have a disproportionate share of health personnel (with the exception of veterinarians – a typically rural occupation). The most urban of the medical occupations are the dentists; they have an association of their own, in addition to the *Colegio de Médicos* (Medical Association), thereby having a double professional control over their members. The least urban medical occupations are *practicantes* (medical assistants), and pharmacists who perform the physician's role in small and medium size towns and in rural areas. Around 36 per cent of the population live in the provincial capitals, which contain 66 per cent of the physicians. This percentage is even higher in the case of specialists: psychiatrists 82 per cent, surgeons 80 per cent, ophthalmologists 76 per cent, pediatricians 70 per cent and gynaecologists 69 per cent. Madrid concentrates all types of health personnel, with its health personnel/population rates reaching double the national average.

Generally speaking, there is no shortage of physicians in Spain, although there are shortages of specialists, particularly dentists and psychiatrists. General practitioners are still more than a third of the total number of physicians, although, as in other southern European countries, their numbers are in decline. In Spain the proportion of GPs is decreasing slowly: in 1956 they constituted 49 per cent of physicians, and in 1970 they had fallen to 43 per cent. In absolute figures the number of GPs is still growing (see Table 1) but at a lower speed than the pediatricians (a specialty in which Spain is relatively well equipped) and psychiatrists.

TABLE 1 Evolution of the number of Physicians in Spain (per 100,000 population)

Years:	Total Physicians	General Practitioners[a]	Pediatry[b]	Surgery[c]	Gynaecology[d]	Psychiatry
1976	151	66.6	13.0	13.2	8.0	4.7
1970	129	56.7	11.9	10.8	7.7	3.4
1966	120	52.9	10.8	10.0	7.6	2.6
1960	114	53.8	8.7	8.9	7.2	2.2
1956	106	52.5	7.3	7.9	6.7	2.0

Source: Data from the UMFE (*Unión Médica Farmacéutica Española*).
Notes: [a]*Medicina general.*
[b]*Pediatría* and *Puericultura.*
[c]*Cirugía* and *Traumatismo.*
[d]*Toco-Ginecología.*

Health manpower is concentrated at the university level of education, lacking intermediate and lower levels. If we compare Spain with Yugoslavia in 1970, the disequilibrium is clear:

TABLE 2 Total Health Manpower (per 100,000 population)

	Spain:	Yugoslavia:
University level	213.9	153.3
High level	12.2	187.1
Intermediate level	67.0	158.6
	293.1	499.0

Italy presents an intermediate pattern with a relatively high proportion of health manpower with a university education, but this is not as extreme as the Spanish case. Within the medical profession, psychiatry seems the most underdeveloped sector, but there is a general lack of data about this area. The main shortages are concentrated in the middle-level health occupations, chiefly nursing. If we compare Spain with other southern European countries the lack of a developed nursing profession is striking. This, of course, reflects the general exclusion of women from labour force participation in comparison with socialist or democratic capitalist societies. In summary, the Spanish health manpower structure is lacking low level occupations, even in public hospitals, while the number of physicians is relatively high for the stage of economic development of the country. This distribution concentrates the decision-making power in the hands of the physicians who outnumber the rest of the health manpower population.

In Europe, the relationship between the number of physicians and the number of beds in health establishments is: the poorer or less democratic the country is, the smaller the proportion of beds per doctor it has. This rule is not always applicable to individual countries, but the tendency is. The southern European countries (Figure 2) have fewer beds per physician than the rest of Europe. Spain has the smallest number of beds per doctor in Europe. This suggests both a low standard of services and an imbalance in the distribution of health manpower. The lack of beds and associated hardware and the lack of paramedical staff mean that much medical practice will be at a relatively lower technical level than in the capitalist democracies of northern Europe, as can be seen in the poor ECFMG performance of Spanish doctors.

In this field too, there are pronounced regional variations, which identify three groups of provinces: (1) a set of provinces with low rates of both physicians and hospital beds: mainly Andalusian provinces (without a local medical school), Estremadura and Galicia, being the poorest regions of Spain; (2) a set of provinces that have relatively more physicians than hospital beds, and that are almost exclusively the provinces with medical schools; and (3) a third group of provinces with low rates of physicians but high rates of hospital beds; those are provinces around other well-developed provinces: Guadalajara, Alava, Tarragona, Gerona, Palencia, Teruel, etc. and their hospitals serve the developed provinces.

Other than in socialist or social democratic countries, two systems of health service can usually be found: a public system that attends workers and the poor and a private system for the middle and upper classes. However, in Spain, the urban upper classes utilise both the socialised and private health services. In Spain, as in other capitalist countries, the private health care system tends to concentrate on curative treatment, leaving preventive and rehabilitative work in public hands. This is due to the lack of a national health service financed by the national budget, and the profit orientation of the profession. The Spanish health system shows a slight tendency towards socialisation.

Figure 2 Hospital Beds per Physician in Europe 1970

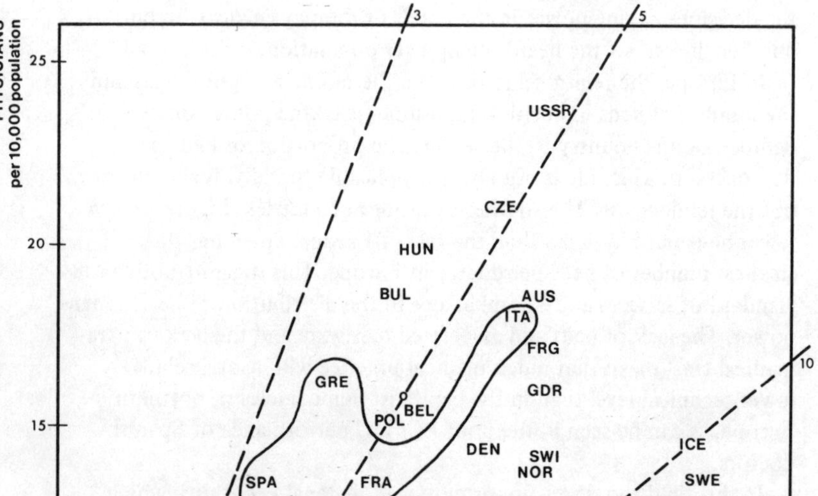

Source: WHO, *World Health Annual 1970*, vol. 3, pp. 121-22, 224-5.

This situation creates many problems for the medical profession which works both in public and private organisations. At present over 70 per cent of physicians work (at least part time) for the *Seguro de Enfermedad* which is the national health insurance system that covers 90 per cent of the population, including outpatient care and hospitalisation, but excluding mental health services and a part of the rural population. This trend is changing the situation of the medical profession, which is more dependent each year on the public administration.

A notable feature of health care organisation in Spain is the (relative) lack of political power of the medical profession in relation to their colleagues in other countries. None of Franco's ministers – out of a list of more than one hundred – was a physician. As a consequence of the lack of power, the prestige of the medical profession is also lower. The (relative) lack of prestige is compensated for by the accumulation of wealth through the multiple jobs held by most physicians.[5] This is common practice in three situations which cover most Spanish doctors: (1) where the doctor's family is upper class with extensive business interests; (2) where medical services are insufficiently developed to support a doctor at the economic level he expects, (3) where the doctor's family is based in rural areas with extensive local business and farming interests and the local population is too sparse or too poor to support a doctor economically.

Spain is also notable for the low participation of women in the medical labour force: In 1968, only 3.5 per cent of physicians were women, probably one of the lowest proportions (if not the lowest) in Europe. The low participation of women in the labour force is a problem that Spain has tried to face in recent years with little apparent success. A recognised problem among female medical students is that a high percentage of them do not practise medicine after graduation. In a country where the state is confessional – Roman Catholic in the case of Spain – the medical profession services as a means of social control on issues such as abortion, birth control, sexual attitudes, delivery patterns, illegitimacy and mental illness. This control presses most upon the lower classes who have less education, fewer resources and necessarily have to use the public services.

For a long time the physician's role has been that of adapting individuals to their environment. In the case of non-democratic countries this means a greater effort is made to control the population. These features are stressed when the country has a capitalist and dependent economy, as well as an established Roman Catholic church, as is the case of Spain. On the other hand, democratic countries are accepting more and more that the role of the physicians should be that of adapting the environment to the lives of individuals.[6] The position of socialist countries is rather ambivalent in this respect: in general, they give greater prominence to preventive measures in relation to physical health, although other aspects of their practice may amount to crude attempts to mould individuals to an environment.

The Ideology of Spanish Physicians

Ideology, in its origins, meant a way of translating ideas into action. At present it is commonly used with the connotation of a socio-political programme. Ideology is a pattern of thought, or an organised system of opinions, beliefs or values about society and life.[7] Including 'ideology' in the analysis of the role of the medical profession is, as I am aware, an ideological definition *per se*. From a Marxian point of view, social structure determines both consciousness and knowledge, as well as ideology.[8] An ideology does not need to be proven as a reality but only believed, although it may, of course, express truths. What is important in the analysis of ideology is not its content (it does not matter if this refers to true or false explanations of life) but the interests behind its formulation.

There are several groups in society which are granted the legitimate use of ideology including the church, politicians and medical doctors. In the case of the medical profession the ideology is a set of beliefs and values about human beings and society held by the profession as a justification of both its actions (autonomy and monopoly) and its manifest goals as a group. The distinctive feature of the ideology of the medical profession is its use in the competition for control over certain areas of personal and social life (body, illness, death) with other institutions (church, economic circles). Ideology in this context legitimises medical authority. In addition, it plays the role of integrating the medical profession in common policies, attitudes or beliefs.

Health ideologies are common precisely because the term 'health' is unclear and has many value connotations. Although we could use texts from a single Spanish author to describe the content of an ideology, we are not interested in individual versions, other than as examples of a group's system of beliefs. Socialisation into the medical ideology is a complicated process. It is supported in Spain by three factors; the length of medical training, the fact that many medical students' parents are physicians, and, in general, the fact that medical students tend to come from higher social class backgrounds than students in other professions.

Ideology is usually considered in singular terms, as it includes a total view of society and life. Nevertheless, there can be differences, even contradictions, between sub-ideologies. 'The medical ideology, like other ideologies, is not a neatly articulated web of mutually compatible statements. Some inconsistent strands do exist, and may make the observer wonder how the medical profession and the individual physician can hold such incompatible, and sometimes opposing premises.'[9] Within the medical ideology we can detect several sub-ideologies. A study of all the opinions, attitudes and behaviour of the medical profession in a country would be a lengthy task. For the present, we have isolated a set of six concrete ideologies which are related to the whole society.[10] In the case of Spain some of the most important sub-ideologies to analyse are: (1) the defence of a race and feelings of nationalism; (2) the defence and justification of the Roman Catholic Church; (3) the fight against a rational way of controlling natality (birth control, abortion); (4) the opposition to the socialisation of the health services and medical careers; (5) the use of medical authority to oppose the rights of minorities (the poor, women); (6) the role of the medical profession as a means of social control in reference to illness, mental disturbance and other deviant cases. There are dissonances among these sub-ideologies, but in general they are consistent; for example, the defence of the Roman Catholic Church and the opposition to birth control measures or the sexual education of the population. The latter is consistent with the sexist approach of medical practice, and the protection of a high birth rate, which in turn favours the imperialist goals of Spain.

In Spain the topics of race and natalist ideology correspond to the imperialist political attitudes of Franco's regime. A paradigmatic example of this attitude is evident in the following quote: 'We cannot conceive of health as a profession, but rather as a mission, in which service and sacrifice will have the enormous reward of the feeling of collaboration with the creating effort of an Empire.'[11] In a similar line, Alfonso de la Fuente, president of the Spanish medical association, and a well-known rightist said in 1942: 'Our health unity is politically, historically and religiously rooted in our way of life; it is written on the millenarian stones of our temples and in the bloody trenches of our Revolution [the Spanish Civil War, 1936-39].'[12] But explicit references to a superior *race* are scarce in the medical literature. Our example of this approach can be found in Agustín Aznar writing in 1942 about physical education: 'With sports the Falange attempts to benefit man and achieve a racial betterment by ruling and leading physical exercise, fighting against the organic defects of this imperial race that has amazed the world with its physical resistance, not only in the burning and arid deserts of Morocco, but also in the frozen Russian steppes.'[13]

An ideology does not only tell us how the world is, but how the world should be. In the medical profession this is frequently the case as many of the beliefs relate to moral, religious and ethical questions. The more traditional and religious a region is, the more important is the role of the medical ideology over ethical and moral issues, and the less important are the scientific characteristics of the profession. In the case of Spain that defence of the Roman Catholic Church goes to the extreme of seriously identifying the physician with the priest.[14] Being an officially recognised Roman Catholic country the medical profession is closely related to the religious orders, and it serves many times as the religious gatekeeper. This structure tends to redefine the classical patient role features,[15] as well as the organisation of health services.[16] There is a cultural pattern that remains to be studied: Catholic ideology at the beginning of this century advised doctors to save the baby's life before that of the mother. As the country developed economically, maternal morality from pregnancy or birth decreased, while the new-born mortality rate increased.

Both society and the medical profession tend to define ways in which people should control their lives. During the last decades Spain has favoured a high birth rate for the following reason: 'There is no Empire, without increasing and spiritualising the national demographic index; and it will not increase without giving back to the rural areas its creative potentiality and overflowing vitality. The Health organisation is the nexus of union through which the rural areas, the permanent nursery of Spain, may forge the Empire.'[17] Botella Llusiá, eminent Spanish gynaecologist, and former *Rector* (President) of the University of Madrid, defended the natalist ideology in the following terms: 'The reasons why it is necessary [to have] a larger amount of children for the Country, are obvious. We should remember that the countries with a rapid and continuous increment of population are those which sooner or later end up imposing themselves on others, and triumphing in the world.'[18]

Ideology may not coincide with reality but still has a coherent existence. For example, the birth control behaviour of the Spanish population is very different from the ideology of the medical profession, although this profession is responsible for supplying birth control devices.[19] In the case of Spain the anti-birth control ideology was the official policy of the government under the influence of the *Opus Dei* and its technocratic leadership in the sixties.[20]

In Spain abortion is prohibited (except in extreme cases to save the life of the mother), and legislation was passed against publicising methods of birth control or the sale of contraceptive materials. Doctors have never had any formal training in these matters. In 1973 the *Real Academia de Medicina,* using inaccurate data, officially condemned abortion, 'The interruption of pregnancy by an artificial method, even under medical control and in a well equipped hospital, has a high incidence of complications. Also maternal mortality in these cases is not negligible.'[21] Abortion – according to this institution – has dangerous consequences for the world population: decline of natality and secondary sterility.

The medical profession in Spain is usually opposed to the reorganisation of medical care, and an effective socialisation of medicine. Physicians are always preoccupied with the increasing number of medical students that might reduce (relatively) their power and monopoly. However, the profession opposed the creation of the national health service (the SOE) with little success. The president of one provincial medical association in Spain, Dr Quesada Sanz, explained that this opposition was based on the reduction of the number of the population attended by private practitioners, and also the poverty and unemployment of many physicians together with the proletarianisation of the medical profession.[22] A characteristic of the Spanish medical profession is its limited power in the area of medical organisation and lack of participation in the formulation of health policies. Decisions within the Spanish medical profession are usually taken by physicians who do not practice, although the patient-physician relationship is used as a criterion to legitimise the autonomy and monopoly of the profession.

The relationship between the physician and the patient is typically authoritarian. The idea is that the patient must be subservient to the orders of the physicians and not bother him (usually *him*) with questions. In general, the patient is not informed about his medical problems. This happens in a higher degree in the national health insurance system (SOE) where the social differences between physician and patient are greater. Authoritarianism is reflected in the sexual education of the population and the sexist approach. Sexual education according to a Spanish medical school textbook consists of the following: 'to inform about the sexual organs, sexual life, fecundation, pregnancy, delivery, etc. insisting that chastity is always commendable to single persons, and premarital sexual contacts always censured'.[23] One of the most influential gynaecologists in Spain said in 1973: 'There are many women, including mothers of numerous children, that confess not to have had, or on rare occasions, sexual pleasure; nevertheless, they are not frustrated by this, because women, even though they may say otherwise, what they look for in a man is motherhood . . . sometimes I have thought that women are physiologically frigid.'[24] Both the advice and treatment given to women tend to be authoritarian, sexist and patriarchal with the implicit purpose of keeping women out of a power position, and to keep them working as housewives or as a low-wage labour force. A characteristic attitude found in a scholarly study on the SOE, is the following:

> At the base of these factors determinant of morbidity it is fitting to place the new social structure provoked by women's working outside their homes, because these factors are not translated exclusively by the deprivations, excesses and anxieties which manifest themselves in the health of the working woman, bur rather they act as a motive for the disintegration of the family, associated with a lack of care for early infancy, hygienic surveillance of children and adolescents, physiological protection and mental formation. Work by females produces an inclination towards independence with a neglect of motherhood, but even when this neglect is overcome, there are defective gestations, which later appear as hereditary handicaps, since during the last few months of pregnancy a woman is incapable of doing heavy work.[25]

The medical profession does not only apply its methods of social control to diseases and patients but uses it also in a broader social scene. This has been recognised by social scientists of all ideologies, from Parsons to Berlinguer.[26] Speaking of the medical schools in Portugal before 1974, for example, Miller Guerra, a well-known physician from the faculty of the Medical School at Lisbon suggested: 'We are aware that university institutions are normally conservative and – so many times! – reactionary. Instead of being, as it is believed, an instrument or incentive of social and intellectual transformations, they oppose change.' The use of mental hospitals as institutions for the detention of deviants is a clear example of the use of medical ideology with the goal of social control. In recent years this has become recognised and led to a move towards replacing detention by increasing the facilities for outpatient treatment, day hospitals and community services for mentally disturbed patients. This trend is still very weak in

Spain.

Power and Conflicts

The Spanish medical profession has usually played the role of slowing down reform, opposing health measures which may decrease its power or control its private practice. The medical profession combines private practice with part-time work in the national health service organisations, mixing resources and the utilisation of equipment. On many occasion drugs and hospital care for private patients have been paid by the social security administration, as a consequence of this double role of the medical profession.

The medical profession enjoys more freedom to define its structure and attitudes toward change than many other groups in society. However, this profession opposes change more strongly than other social groups. In Spain, the medical profession has resisted any change towards a more rational health organisation by appealing to élitist reasons of quality of medical research and care of well-to-do minorities.[27] In its conservatism it represents the convergence of two of the most traditional sectors of society; health and education. It is not surprising that the education of medical students in Spain does not stress team work, independent thinking or critical judgement. But the conservative role of the medical profession in Spain is not a direct consequence of the non-democratic features of the country, as is shown by a comparison with the role of Portuguese doctors before the revolution.[28] The main difference is the existence of a large bourgeoisie off which the Spanish medical profession has lived. The combination of a capitalist and a non-democratic country makes the medical profession less interested in social change.

In our view, in a non-democratic country, based on a capitalistic structure, the health sector is forced to the lowest position on the scale of resources and expenses. Planning tends to be more 'economic' than 'social'. If there is no middle class that can support the medical profession, the latter suffer numerous strains, that may crystallise in the socialisation of health services (the case of Spain), or the socialisation of the whole society if it is added to similar situations in other sectors (Portugal in 1974). When this does not occur, and the system still remains centralised, there is only one exit: the degradation of the health status of the population, and the proliferation of communicable diseases and all other kinds of illnesses. An underdeveloped region or country with a socialised structure will not face this problem of a market-without-resources, but the quality of health services will probably remain low while the country is developing. In non-democratic countries the medical profession has less power, as it competes with other social groups which do not need to legitimise their power. In this case, the influence of the medical profession based on charismatic-humanitarian features is much lower, especially as the authoritarian-totalitarian state does not allow the creation of strong associations, even professional ones. As a consequence, the medical profession is divided into two groups: the opposition which has very little power both as profession and as citizens, and the loyal group of physicians that play the legitimising role. The diffusion of conservative ideologies is the new role of the medical profession in those countries, whereas in democratic countries this role is less important.

Usually, the regional health disequilibria are analysed as a typical problem of economic development, even in Spain where the differences are extreme. This focus ignores the fact that the most pressing health differences are in the end political problems, that is, of social classes and allocation of power. Most of the regional inadequacies in health manpower organisation and distribution have been due to the slight influence of regions in the national health planning processes. This is also the opinion of the World Health Organisation:

> Regional development programmes were usually undertaken on the initiative of the central authorities. Consequently, they might be imperfectly adapted to the actual regional situation unless there was participation of the population and services in the region. Unfortunately, this participation, even when present, was usually restricted or purely advisory and lacking in effective responsibility.[29]

Regional problems in health manpower are aggravated by the lack of autonomy of local and regional communities, that is to say the lack of democracy at a regional level. This problem is obvious in Spain due to the enormous internal migration trends (even compared to other southern European countries), and the increasing nationalism of Catalonia and the Basque country (the two most developed regions).

Competition within the medical profession is high, and is not based on merit but on particularism. This situation creates a generation gap within the profession, which pushes some young doctors to emigrate. The percentage of candidates that passes the 'foreign' (ECFMG) examination is inferior to the world average. This fact stresses the low quality of the medical education in Spain, which is in the hands of the older generation of physicians. In conclusion, it can be suspected that the poor quality of the medical schools in Spain is partially sustained by the established profession which tries to diminish the competition.

Physicians in Spain are usually playing two roles: (1) the role of the private practitioner with a bourgeois clientele which pays high fees; and (2) the physician working part time in a public hospital from which he selects his private clientele. Even when more than 80 per cent of the population is insured by the *Seguro de Enfermedad*, less than a third of housewives answered (in a national sample in 1970) that they would call a physician from the *Seguro de Enfermedad* in case of an emergency. This percentage is even lower in Madrid (26 per cent) where it functions well in comparison to the rest of Spain.

In summary, the health manpower in non-democratic countries accomplishes at least three different tasks: (1) the protection of private interests in order to assure medicine as a profiteering occupation and a good business for the private sector; (2) an instrument for the justification of the political regime as well as the diffusion of both social and political ideologies; and (3) a structure to oppose class, urban or regional redistribution, and other revolutionary changes.

Notes

1. This is similar to the concept of 'health system', that is to say: 'the set of relationships among institutions, social groups, and individuals that is directed toward maintaining and improving the health status of a certain human population'. J.M. de Miguel, 'A framework for the study of national health systems'. Inquiry supplement to vol. 12, no. 2 (June 1975), p. 13. However, the health systems of non-democratic countries may accomplish other latent functions (power legitimation, international loans, propaganda).
2. Eliot Freidson, *Profession of Medicine* (New York: Dodd, Mead and Co., 1972); Samuel W. Bloom, *The Doctor and His Patient* (New York: The Free Press, 1965); Everett C. Hughes *et al., Twenty Thousand Nurses Tell Their Story* (Philadelphia: J.B. Lippincott, 1958).
3. Bui-Dang-Ha Doan, 'World trends in medical manpower: 1950-1970'. *World Health Statistics Report*, vol. 27, no. 2 (1974), p. 92.
4. In Spain the number of physicians reflects those registered in the provincial *Colegios Medicos,* the only ones allowed to practice with the exception of those in the military hospitals and the physicians of the *Cuerpo Nacional de Sanidad* (public health officers).
5. There are several ways of exploiting patients: *Dico* is the abbreviation of 'dichotomy' which refers to the custom of dividing the patient's bill between the general practitioner (usually 40 per cent) and the specialist. This is done, of course, without the knowledge of the patient. *Tarugo* refers to the percentage of profits that the pharmaceutical industry pays to a doctor doctor who writes the prescriptions.
6. This is the opinion of Giovanni Berlinguer in Italy: *Medicina e politica* (Bari: De Donato, 1973), p. 22.

7. Ideology can also be defined as the set of false – or at least distorted – ideas used by a group in order to obtain or maintain power. This is not a complete definition of ideology as it can be a true set of ideas; and power is not the only (although it is the most important) goal of ideology. The second characteristic is even clearer in the case of a medical profession.
8. This idea appears in *German Ideology*, written in 1846:

> 'The phantoms formed in the human brain are also necessarily, sublimates of their material life-process, which is empirically verifiable and bound to material premises. Morality, religion, metaphysics, all the rest of ideology and their corresponding forms of consciousness, thus no longer retain the semblance of independence. They have no history, no development; but men, developing their material production and their material intercourse, alter, along with this real existence, their thinking. Life is not determined by consciousness, but consciousness by life.

9. Bernard R. Blishen, *Doctors and Doctrines: The Ideology of Medical Care in Canada* (Toronto: University of Toronto Press, 1969), p. 140.
10. For a study of opinions and ideologies of the Spanish medical profession, see Amando de Miguel, 'La profesión médica en España'. *Papers: Revista de Sociología* 5 (1976).
11. Words of Agustín Aznar, *delegado nacional de sanidad,* in his article: 'La sanidad como misión'. *Ser* 6 (1942), p.10.
12. Alfonso de la Fuente, 'Rutas de la unidad sanitaria'. *Ser* 3 (1942), p. 4.
13. Agustín Aznar, 'La sanidad . . . ' op. cit., p. 10.
14. About the concept of the religious character of the patient-physician relationship see Pedro Laín Entralgo, 'La estructura de la relación entre el médico y el enfermo'. Pp. 111-123 in Thure Von Vexkull *et al.* (eds)., *Medicina y Sociedad. Revista de la Universidad de Madrid*, vol. 10, no. 37 (1961), pp. 122-3.
15. 'The Judeo-Christian religion contains numerous incentives to being ill or disabled. States of distress and failure – whether because of stupidity, poverty, sickness, or what not – may be interpreted as potentially desirable goals, for as the hungry infant is given the mother's breast, so the disabled human being is promised God's all-embracing helpfulness and benevolence. This pattern of human interaction and communication is regarded as the main source of a vast number of rules, all of which conspire, as it were, to foster man's infantilism and dependence.' Thomas S. Szasz, *The Myth of Mental Illness: Essays on the Psychiatric Dehumanization of Man* (Garden City, N.Y.: Doubleday, 1961), p. 303.
16. For example, the names of the hospitals in Spain keep a religious affiliation. In Barcelona about 43 per cent of hospitals in 1970 had a religious name, in comparison to 35 per cent in Madrid. (On the one hand only 1 per cent of hospitals in Barcelona had a political name in comparison to 7 per cent in Madrid.) Some of the religious names imply sufferings and unhappiness: *Clínica del Remedio, Clínica de la Milagrosa, Sanatorio Virgen del Recuerdo S.A. Hospital de Nuestra Señora de la Esperanza, Hospital Casa de Caridad de San Lázaro, Hospital de las Colonias Extranjeras Enfermería Evangelica.*
17. Alfonso de la Fuente, 'La sanidad en el medio rural '. *Ser* 4 (1942), p. 3.
18. Jose Botella Llusiá, *Reproducción y demografía* (Madrid: Revista de la Universidad de Madrid, 1944), p. 47.
19. Traditional methods of controlling fertility in Spain were: late marriage, prostitution, sexual attitudes, prolonged lactation, control over sexual

freedom, abstinence at certain times (Holy Week and Lent, menstrual periods, before marriage).

20. An example of this ideology can be seen in a book by the professor of the University of Navarre, Manuel Ferrer Regales (1972). The author is scandalised by the 'progressive sexual freedom, that in honour of a supposed women's liberation and following a development of the erotic, stresses the anti-natalist mentality in millions of people' (p.25).
21. See the *Boletín Informativo del Consejo General de Colegios Médicos,* the official publication of the Spanish Medical Association.
22. Jesús Quesada Sanz, *El Seguro de Enfermedad y los médicos en el momento actual* (n.p.: Imprenta el Tiempo, 1962), pp. 5 ff.
23. Gonzalo Piédrola, 'Higiene individual' pp. 599-614 in J. Balén *et al.* (eds.), *Medicina preventiva y social, Higiene* (Madrid: Amaro, 1971), p. 609.
24. See the declarations of Botella Llusiá, in an interview in *Tauta* 14 (1973), p. 609.
25. Enrique Serrano, *El seguro de enfermedad y sus problemas* (Madrid: Instituto de Estudios Politicos, 1950), pp. 22-3.
26. Talcott Parsons, *The Social System* (New York: The Free Press, 1951); Giovanni Berlinguer, *Medicina e politica* (Bari: De Donato, 1973). A provocative analysis of the medical profession as a system of social control can be seen in Barbara Ehrenreich and John Ehrenreich, 'Social control functions of the medical system'. *Health Politics* vol. 4, no. 2 (1974), pp. 19-24. In *Ideology and Insanity*, Szasz has pointed out that psychoanalysis began as a critique of the psychiagric ideology, to be soon coopted by the medical ideology (New York: Dell Pu. Co., 1970), pp. 69-78.
27. One expert on health matters, interviewed in a Mediterranean country – in 1972 – expressed the following opinion:

    You can talk about health being a privilege or a right. We can not call it a right in . . . [the country] because that will mean that everybody has to be given the same health services. We do not have resources for this. It is not possible because medical doctors do not want to go to rural areas. For us health is a privilege. The problem is not only with health, you could say the same thing about education, etc. In a system such as ours it is obvious that those who have money can buy better health services.

28. The Portuguese medical profession has been one of the most important factors advocating health reform in the country; it has been a basic proponent of change towards a global health reform in the sixties. The reasons are various: the relationships of the medical profession with the regimes of Salazar and Caetano; the poor economic situation of most of the physicians; the criticism of the *Ordem dos Medicos*; and the influence of specific medical leaders (such as Miller Guerra or Gonçalves Ferreira). The lack of political parties before the revolution allowed both the medical association and the medical leaders to have a considerable importance as health pressure groups. This has decreased with the creation of political parties and the participation of the people in the organisation of health structures.
29. WHO Regional Office for Europe, *The Health Aspects of Planning for Regional Socio-Economic Development* (Copenhagen: WHO, 1968), p. 8.

Eugene Gallagher's discussion of home dialysis and socio-medical policy follows interestingly from de Miguel's paper for, in a specific instance and a quite different society, Gallagher also shows how important are the economic and the political structures for the provision of health care.

He raises two particularly interesting issues. The first has to do with the changes in a dominant pattern of social relations brought about by technological advance; the second with the reasons for the establishment of particular patterns of treatment.

Gallagher shows how the availability of a reasonably reliable life-saving technology, too expensive for most patients to afford, led to U.S. federal funding for all. This was a break in the pattern whereby such aid had been restricted to the poor and the old. At the same time the locus of treatment has tended to change, so that while at the outset home dialysis was extolled as being better for the patient in terms of autonomy, morale and rehabilitation than centre dialysis, the trend is now away from the home to the centre. Now only 25 per cent of patients dialyse at home while 37 per cent did formerly and it is estimated that 50 per cent could. Moreover home dialysis is thought to be 40 per cent cheaper than institutional dialysis. Since the programme, at $331 million in 1975, was 60 per cent higher than expected, there is federal pressure to encourage home dialysis, a pressure which is resisted by the medical profession.

In explaining the trend, Gallagher is inclined to emphasise the strain upon familial relations which home dialysis involves and upon the patient in terms of costs of materials and the labour of machine maintenance. He also gives weight to the changing characteristics of the patients who now include more elderly and more disadvantaged among the 19,000 currently maintained, compared with the privileged 300 of 1964.

At the same time his analysis makes plain that there are some interests vested in centre analysis, not least the non-hospital-based profit making dialysis centres. Centre dialysis also relieves the renal specialist of detailed involvement with the process, since trained technicians take day-to-day responsibility, technicians who are not available to the patient at home. For patients at a distance from a renal specialist home dialysis must also depend on the willingness of the community physician to accept training. Thus complex problems in the division of labour, including the patient's own labour, are clearly involved. Whether the trend to the centre is in the best interests of the patients or of others remains unresolved.

M.S.

HOME DIALYSIS AND SOCIOMEDICAL POLICY

Eugene B. Gallagher

Health care is increasingly a governmental responsibility in modern societies. Medical sociology can contribute to a rational analysis of political, economic and administrative issues in the formation and implementation of governmental health policy. The basic idea in this paper is that, under the impetus of the traditional humane ethic of medicine and a modern technological imperative 'to do everything possible', the health care system and government of contemporary societies attempt to provide renal dialysis to all patients who need it. From this idea flow many consequences and implications of interest to the medical sociologist, regarding the processes by which health policy is determined and implemented in society, resource allocation in health care, and the microdynamics of the relationships between the dialysis patient, his physician and his family.

Renal dialysis has several features which make it a therapy of particular interest to medical sociologists. Chronic renal failure requires dialysis as a lifelong therapy (unless the patient receives a transplant). With proper training and supportive family circumstances, the patient can carry out dialysis in his home – although dialysis is a very exacting 'high technology' form of treatment. Economic considerations recommend home dialysis, and there may be additional, less tangible benefits to the patient in the form of greater autonomy, morale and rehabilitation. These aspects of home dialysis in turn link up with questions concerning the allocation and effectiveness of treatment resources.

In the United States, an extensive mobilisation of dialysis resources has occurred because of recent (1972) federal legislation which pays for the treatment. This legislation has been hailed by some observers as a model for a future programme of national health insurance which would underwrite the expense of designated catastrophic illnesses, rather than illness in general. Opponents of such an approach wrote a report highly critical of the recent legislation ironically entitled 'Disease by Disease Toward National Health Insurance?' (Institute of Medicine, 1973). The legislation and the ensuing controversy over it illustrate the tension, especially strong in the United States, between categorical and comprehensive approaches to health care. By receiving a categorical designation, chronic renal failure became a 'policy disease'. It will be useful now to review the technological developments leading to this categorical status.

Much Gained but Still a Way to Go: Biomedical Progress Against Renal Failure

The recent history of the treatment of chronic renal failure is a bright chapter in the annals of progress in biomedicine. Apparatus for hemodialysis was developed during the Second World War, and renal transplantation has been performed since 1951. Hemodialysis became available as a long-term therapy when a method of repetitively tapping into the patient's blood circulation was developed in 1960.

A simplified sketch of current therapy for the patient is as follows. As renal function declines, the patient produces less urine and that urine which is produced contains fewer waste products filtered by the kidneys from the blood circulation. The patient becomes uremic, i.e. urea accumulates in the blood. Without relief, the uremic patient will expire in one or two weeks. Dialysis rescues him; the dialysis patient has been aptly described as 'intermittently dying' (Beavert, 1974).

In the process of hemodialysis, the patient's blood is pumped through a dialyser. The dialyser contains a large membrane surface and a biochemically-composed solution, or dialysate. The patient's blood flows on one side of the membrane and the dialysate on the other side. Processes of osmosis and filtration occur, by which the patient's blood is 'cleansed' of urea and its electrolyte balance maintained in an approximation of natural kidney function.

Varying with the type of dialyser used and his or her blood volume, a patient is dialysed for about twenty-four hours a week, in two or three separate sessions. For each session, it is necessary to set up the equipment and dialysate, and then to dismantle and clean it – a time-consuming routine. Between sessions, the patient must adhere to a stringent diet, the most difficult part of which is probably the drastic restriction on fluid intake. In addition to maintaining blood composition, the natural kidney performs more complex functions, pertaining to regulation of blood pressure, bone metabolism and growth in children, which are not duplicated by dialysis. Thus, over an extended time period, the dialysis patient may experience medical difficulties and require additional treatment beyond dialysis.

Efforts are under way to perfect a portable dialyser which the patient can wear. This would obviate the need for programmed sessions with the dialysis machine and permit a relaxation of dietary rigours.

Renal transplantation, by providing the chronic renal failure victim with a natural kidney, is a more adequate replacement therapy than dialysis. The difficulty with it, however, is unless the transplanted kidney is a good histological match, the recipient's immunological system will reject it. For this reason, transplant recipients take steroid drugs indefinitely to suppress the immune reaction. Although the transplant recipient is spared the burdens of diet and dialysis sessions, the immunosuppressive régime renders him more vulnerable to infection and to undesirable side effects.

The mortality rate among renal patients remains high. The investment of time, energy and motivation necessary to sustain life on dialysis is large, indeed daunting to outsiders when they are initiated into 'renal culture'. Yet the success stories of dialysis patients carrying out normal family, work and community roles, are also quite outstanding.

In this paper I will deal with dialysis only and will focus upon recent changes in health policy in the United States regarding renal dialysis.

Chronic Renal Failure as a Policy Disease

An important index of the acceptability of renal failure technology, not only to patients and doctors, but to American society at large is the federal programme of financial support for treatment of End-Stage Renal Disease (ESRD), starting in June 1973. Social equity in access to health care is one desideratum which most people would regard as a valuable goal. Progressiveness is another: how rapidly and how broadly can a health care system assess and implement the advances produced by biomedical research? The enactment of the Medicaid (for the poor) and the Medicare (for the elderly, who tend also to be poor) programmes of payment of health services had moved American society some distance towards equalising access to health care while maintaining physician autonomy and fee-for-service. The federal ESRD programme can be seen, in the most favourable light, as an attempt at the simultaneous maximisation of both equity and progressiveness.

There was much publicity about transplantation and dialysis, and about the plight of patients facing death unless they could pay for treatment during the 1960s. In smaller communities, campaigns were organised to meet transplantation expenses, or to purchase dialysis equipment for a local renal victim. National organisations became active. The National Kidney Foundation, which had been organised earlier to promote research into renal disease, became concerned also with access to treatment for renal patients. The National Association of

Patients on Hemodialysis and Transplantation (NAPHT) was formed as a lay organisation to develop a community of interest and enhance the life-chances of renal patients. Several analytical studies commissioned or conducted by the federal government assayed the total medical, economic and social dimensions of renal failure as a national public health problem and offered recommendations for the deployment of dialysis and transplation resources, in anticipation of later federal funding (Burton, 1967; Hallan *et al.*, 1968; LeSourd *et al.*, 1968).

These various developments served as a prelude to the enactment by the U.S. Congress of the financial support legislation. Although the legislation had many friends and few enemies, it was introduced and passed by an oblique strategy. In the Senate, Senators Hartke of Indiana and Long of Louisiana introduced a bill to designate ESRD as a disability which would entitle the patient to coverage under the Federal Social Security-Medicare social insurance programme. This coverage was to be extended to all ages; it was not to be confined to persons aged sixty-five and over, as in the Medicare legislation of 1965. Moreover, it was to cover not only the working population which directly contributes to Social Security-Medicare insurance, but also their spouses and other dependents, roughly 90 per cent of the American population. The amendment preserved the same co-payment feature which was incorporated earlier into Medicare: 80 per cent payment by the federal government and 20 per cent by the patient (or his private insurance or other payer).

Technically, the Hartke-Long proposal was an amendment to the Social Security Act of 1972. In support of his bill, Senator Hartke read into the *Congressional Record* a *New York Times* article by Lawrence Altman which described the pioneering efforts of the Northwest Kidney Center in the state of Washington to extend dialysis treatment to virtually all victims in the metropolitan Seattle area (Altman, 1971). Altman's article described the situation of Ernie Crowfeather, a part-Indian native of Washington, who was both a convicted robber and a renal failure patient. Ernie's situation dramatised the argument that Senator Hartke urged upon the Senate: an affluent, technologically-advanced society was morally obliged not to restrict life-saving treatment to the most worthy renal victims but to all in need, even to criminals. He estimated the cost of the programme at $75 million the first year, rising to $250 million after four years.

Senators Magnuson and Jackson of Washington endorsed the amendment, and Senator Dole of Kansas made two points: first, that he had lived the past twenty-five years with only one kidney and second, that he supported the amendment although it singled out one disease only for financial help. Senator Bennett of Utah opposed it because other, equally important, health care problems were ignored. In the brief debate no one specifically challenged the figures which Senator Hartke projected for the cost of the programme and which later turned out to be a serious underestimate. There was no discussion either of the broadened Medicare eligibility or of the proposed administration of the programme. The Senate approved the Hartke-Long proposal 52-3, with 45 senators not present or not voting.

The amendment was approved by the House of Representatives as part of the total Social Security bill, without separate attention. It became law 30 October 1972, to go into effect in July 1973. With that, renal failure became a 'policy disease', lifting it out of the fellowship of heart disease, cancer, diabetes and other serious ills and conferring upon it a special status. The availability of a reasonably reliable technology, too expensive for most patients to obtain, prompted government intervention and financial rescue.

Chronic renal failure has several features which make its treatment a good candidate for public financing. It is not primarily a disease of the elderly, particularly when renal failure is the sole medical problem and is not the by-product of diabetes or hypertension. Glomerulonephritis, the disease entity responsible for the greatest amount of renal failure, attacks many patients in youth or middle age, with a resulting toll of untimely disability and death. Much treatment effort is thus directed toward the rehabilitation of patients who are young enough to be self-supporting and to be responsible for the care and support of others. Public funding thus has the aspect of 'maintenance of function' or of 'investment in human capital'.

In contast with cancer, hypertension and heart disease, renal failure has a 'treatment package' which is relatively discrete, i.e. dialysis and/or transplantation.

The high cost of treatment of renal failure has been mentioned as a major factor impelling federal support. It was seen by federal legislators and officials as being too expensive for the private means of most individuals. Now there is concern about whether the aggregate costs are not too high for the government. Medicare renal failure payments during 1975 came to $331 million, which was 60 per cent higher than the estimates for 1975 made in 1973. Estimates in August 1976 project the total cost for 1977 at $597 million. About five sixths of the payments are for dialysis services, with the remaining one sixth for transplantation services. The dialysis programme is under intense scrutiny for points at which economies can be affected.

Home Dialysis

Home hemodialysis started in 1964 in Seattle and Boston, not long after improvements in the dialysis apparatus and in blood access made possible long-term, repetitive maintenance dialysis, as distinct from short-term dialysis for acute renal failure. In those heroic early days, well-described in Renee Fox's and Judith Swazey's book, *The Courage to Fail* (1974), dialysis resources were scarce and had to be stretched. When rationing was accomplished through a formal selection process rather than by happenstance, the selectors were painfully aware that many patients were being abandoned. The selectors were unhappy with their role as life-sparing and life-denying decision-makers. The scarcity factor lay in the small number of professionals who had the know-how to treat renal failure patients by dialysis, and in the scarcity of apparatus. There were a few pioneering nephrologists in a few locations using a few dialysers. The former scarcity of resources became the matrix for hard choices based upon ethical presuppositions about the comparative worth of lives. By opening the door to a broad-scale application of dialysis, the Social Security amendment defused the pressured, intoxicating preoccupations with 'who shall live', but it raised new issues in socio-medical policy.

Now that dialysis is available to most renal failure patients (19,000 patients in the US at present), the issues become more general and policy-oriented, such as the allocation of funds for treatment; the desirable extent of reliance upon economic incentives for the professional and private sectors to mobilize resources; and the maximum public benefit for the funds expended. Dr Belding Scribner and his associates in the Seattle programme wrote an article in 1968 which asserted: 'Being able to accept several patients for home dialysis in lieu of one patient for center dialysis means that it is morally wrong to take on any more patients for center dialysis until all candidates for dialysis in the home have been given a chance' (Fenton, 1968).

The comparative success of home dialysis and institutionally-provided dialysis is an important question. In regard to patient survival, the evidence suggests little difference in home as compared with institutional dialysis in a hospital or a special dialysis centre. Under either mode, about 90 per cent of a patient cohort survives for one year, and 80 per cent for two years (Lowrie, 1973). The survival figures reflect experience with unmatched and unselected populations. No controlled studies have been done because there is probably not enough sheerly scientific interest in what, from the standpoint of a clinical trial, is the *same* biochemical process occurring in two different environmental settings. Furthermore, if a patient encounters difficulty on the home régime, he will usually be shifted to institutional dialysis, lest his condition seriously deteriorate. This is not an infrequent happening.

If the two modes of dialysis are of equal clinical effectiveness, then public policy would support the more economical. Home dialysis is widely regarded as being far less expensive than institutional dialysis. Since the cost of the ESRD programme is growing by annual leaps and bounds within the federal budget, there is acute governmental interest in curbing the cost, and attention naturally focuses on the economy of dialysis performed in the home. How much cheaper is home dialysis, and what accounts for its cost-saving?

The 1974 edition of *Harrison's Principles of Internal Medicine,* an authoritative American text, states:

> Another problem of chronic hemodialysis is its cost, which at present is estimated at $25,000 (range $20,00 to $30,000) per patient per year in hospital centers. 'Satellite-center' dialysis costs range from $10,000 to $20,000 per year. The cost of home dialysis is considerably less, averaging approximately $5,000 per year after the initial investment in equipment. [*Harrison's Principles of Internal Medicine,* 1974, p. 1382. Satellite-center dialysis or simply, center dialysis, is treatment in a facility, usually privately owned, which receives patients on referral from a community hospital or medical centre.]

A sub-committee of the House of Representatives dealt with the question of cost in an October 1975 report (Sub-committee on Oversight, 22 October 1975). This report estimates that the cost for home dialysis is $4,000 to $6,000 per year; for centre dialysis, $14,000 to $20,000 per year; and for hospital dialysis, approximately $30,000 per year. (Though far the most expensive modality, hospital dialysis is not important for aggregate cost control because it is performed on only a small number of patients, where there is an overriding medical necessity.) It is difficult to frame precise comparisons of the cost of home and centre dialysis. Methods of calculating cost vary and the package of service also varies. For example, some dialysis centres employ social workers and nutritionists for services to both centre-dialysed patients and to the home-dialysed patients whose treatment is supervised from these same institutions. The social workers and nutritionists are paid by fixed salary regardless of how much or little service they render to home patients, and the latter are not billed for their services. This practice thus gives a 'too-high' figure for centre dialysis and a 'too-low' figure for home dialysis. Other centres do not employ social workers and nutritionists. Obviously, cost comparisons should be free of such disparate elements. Despite some uncertainty regarding the exact relative costs of home dialysis and centre dialysis, it appears that the home method is cheaper by a factor of 40 per cent or more, even after hidden costs are assessed to it.

One major reason why home dialysis is cheaper is that dialysis, wherever performed, is a labour-intensive process requiring some two to three hours of work before and after each dialysis period. Home dialysis draws upon the unpaid services of lay persons, including the patient himself, but centre dialysis uses the labour of paid professionals.

While home dialysis is less expensive than centre dialysis in monetary cost, it is *more* expensive to the patient in terms of his own out-of-pocket expense. The home patient pays the full cost for a number of items involved in dialysis, such as the water and electricity consumed, and medical supplies including syringes and adhesive tape. He must also pay 20 per cent of the cost of apparatus purchase or rental. These expenses also apply to centre dialysis but are not charged to the patient there. In addition, the 20 per cent overall copayment charge by the centre is usually forgiven if the patient does not have his own private health insurance to cover it. A further expense for the home patient lies in learning dialysis. The tuition is free, but the patient must pay costs of transportation to the training unit. Also, he is not paid for loss of earnings, either his own or those of any helper who may also receive training.

If the specific monetary burdens of home dialysis are the primary deterrent, this could be removed by a change in the law providing for reimbursement of the patient for these items. A still stronger incentive would be to pay the patient and his helpers for their labour, but this might prove so expensive as to obliterate substantially the relative economy of home dialysis. The rehabilitation gains for the patient and his family from self-management of treatment might even be increased by financial compensation for their effort. Whether legislators could be convinced by this argument is dubious. It is in one sense paradoxical that American society, through its legislative processes, lays out great sums of money to prolong the lives of terminal renal patients but then draws back from supporting related measures which might enhance the patients' autonomy or quality of life. Of course, there is a great difference between volunteer unpaid work and paid work; one difference lies, obviously, in the direct economic cost of the latter, but there are further sociological differences less easy to delineate. Richard Titmuss' social philosophy regarding the value of volunteer blood donation (and the corruptibility of paid 'professional' donation) can perhaps be extended to the patient (or his relatives) who performs essential unpaid services, but with the paradox that the beneficiary is not the remote, faceless recipient of a blood donation, but rather the patient himself (Titmuss, 1971). What might be regarded as unpaid 'charitable' service can then be equally regarded as self-interested survival behaviour. While legislators deliberating whether to compensate patients for operating dialysis machines may be primarily interested in the direct economic costs, sociological factors such as these are relevant.

In a broader sense, there are sociological questions of strategy and policy in the articulation of technological, professional resources in health care with existing patterns of family, household and community relationship for the benefit of patients with chronic illness. How far can the affective strengths and adaptive capabilities of kinship ties be marshalled as a kind of 'low' or 'soft' technology in the support of the scientific 'high' or 'hard' medical technology which relieves pain and saves lives? Policy-makers and health planners tend to accept the high medical technology as an objectively fixed (though subject to improvement through research) structure which imposes its 'just' requirements upon the normative structure of lay and family relationships. Moreover, much of what families contribute to the treatment and management of chronic illness in their members is 'free service', an unrationalisable and yet valuable unbudgeted item in reckoning of the administration of health services. The various ways in which the formal structure of health services in a society can enlist family resources depend greatly, of course, upon the pattern of health service organisation and financing which prevails as medical care moves into an era of high technology and chronic illness. The role of social services as a mediator between the somewhat opaque realm of medical technology and the lay world of family-kin relationships is pivotal. In the United States, social services have been poorly developed and largely stigmatised as applicable only to poor people. It will probably prove difficult in the United States to mobilise on a broad scale the potentials of voluntary lay and family support in dealing with chronic illness; there will be greater resort to purchase of the needed services in the marketplace, along with intensive development of specialised roles and techniques for implementing the 'soft' technology which supports the definitive or 'hard' technology.

Physician Compensation for Dialysis Services

A second important aspect of dialysis cost under the federal legislation is the manner and amount of payment for the renal physician. Perhaps the two most critical questions in the general subject of physician compensation are: first, how does the mode and amount of payment affect the doctor-patient relationship? Second, how does the mode and amount of payment affect the type, amount and quality of services rendered by the doctor?

The renal failure patient is a gravely ill person, but dialysis as a routine treatment does not require on-going attention from a physician. Dialysis is an exacting yet highly standard 'machine run' procedure which can be broken down into a series of simple steps, conceptually and operationally. It does not require the complex clinical judgement of a physician on a continuous basis. Patients on home dialysis manage their treatment without benefit of direct medical assistance, although many have the option of 'hot-line' telephone communication with a dialysis centre or hospital. They can generally cope with apparatus malfunctions and with troublesome emergencies such as the clotting of blood in the shunt. I was exposed to a remarkable example of 'intercontinental dialysis supervision' which well illustrates the routinised, componential nature of the process. A London private nephrologist has in his office a telex by which his home dialysis patients in Africa and the Near East communicate with him. He says the entire procedure can be described by thirteen numerical parameters indicating venous pressure, changes in body weight, fluid pressures in the apparatus, dialysate composition and other elements. So long as the patient (and/or his helper) can report these figures, it is not necessary for him to understand or communicate in the English language. It is well recognised that non-emergency needs can arise in dialysis which require medical judgement and performance, such as treating an infection in the shunt area (portal of blood outflow and inflow), the surgical creation of a fistula (induction of a 'short circuit' between an artery and vein, as a method of blood access alternative to a shunt), and dealing with degenerative changes in bone tissue and endocrine function. But these are complications of dialysis rather than the direct dialysis process.

At first, the federal officials responsible for implementing the renal disease law planned not to identify physician services as a distinct component within the dialysis process. However, just before the programme went into effect in June 1973, the Department of Health, Education, and Welfare (HEW) issued a statement which recognised that renal dialysis services 'do need physicians to provide supervisory and on-call services, and that in some cases such a physician does perform a specific, identifiable medical service to a patient in the course of his dialysis, as when a patient goes into shock' (Sub-committee on Health, US House of Representatives, 24 June 1975, p. 10). On this basis, they permitted doctors to make charges to dialysis centres for their supervisory services. These charges were to be accommodated within the overall allowable fee payable to the dialysis centre for each dialysis, not added to it.

Many renal physicians objected strongly to this. They likened their role and services to those which radiologists, pathologists and anaesthetists perform and argued for the corresponding fee-for-service payment. These latter three types of specialists do not have 'their own' patients and provide indirect (though highly essential) services to patients of other physicians, within the general structure of hospital or laboratory functions. In the United States, these specialists have traditionally resisted being paid a salary by hospitals or clinics and have insisted on having their services separately recognised and directly billed to the patient (or third-party payor). The renal physicians advanced the same argument to HEW. At its most strident, this argument asserts that unless the doctor is paid on a fee-for-service basis, the 'doctor-patient relationship' is endangered.

The final scheme established two methods of payment from which the doctor may choose. One method allows the doctor to render a bill to the dialysis facility for particular services he performs for a patient. This is essentially fee-for-service compensation. The second method allows the doctor to charge a flat monthly amount for all medical services which are related to the renal treatment rendered to a patient, whether the patient needs many such services or none at all in a given month. The figure ranges from \$160 to \$240 per month, with an average of \$200 for dialysis centre patients. For home dialysis patients, the average payment is \$140 per month. About 60 per cent of the renal physicians have elected the second method. There is less paper work, and the rate of effective compensation is quite substantial in relation to the amount of time spent. This very popular flat monthly amount is, in effect, a capitation mode of payment. The physician is paid a fixed amount per time unit (a month) for meeting the medical needs of a designated patient.

In the total compass of modes of physician payment, this application of the capitation principle is highly unusual (Roemer, 1972). Capitation systems have typically been used to pay primary care physicians for the basic medical care of large populations of persons in essential good health. In contrast, the renal programme is clearly in the domain of the technological care of seriously ill persons by specialists.

This application of capitation is viewed by some HEW officials not merely as an opportune way of paying for a particular class of medical services, but as an experiment in national catastrophic health insurance, which if successful might be extended to the compensation of specialists in other major illnesses. The point which these officials have in mind in defining renal capitation as a model innovation is certainly not its probable contribution to the total high expenses of the programme. However deplorable the high expense may be, it can be reduced, in principle at least, by recalibrating the monthly payment at a lower level while still retaining the capitation mode. The experimental feature lies in the relation of payment mode to volume of service rendered. It has been suggested in several studies of payment mode, that when physicians are paid by capitation or by salary, the volume of services generated is lower than when payment comes from separate fees for services rendered.

The renal physicians as a group are held in high regard by federal health policy-makers. Behind the promulgation of the capitation plan lay the expectation that the renal physicians would conscientiously render the full measure of services necessary for patient welfare, resisting the normal tendency to cut back once the payment is fixed. On this basis it can be said that the experiment was launched on favourable terms, its success being entrusted to highly specialised physicians who are accustomed to dealing with gravely ill patients on a long-term basis.

One other feature of the arrangement can be drawn, to contrast it with the more familiar capitation support of primary care practitioners. Medical consultants in Great Britain and other countries with a comprehensive health system commonly complain that the capitation-supported primary care doctors refer too many patients to them; the theory is that the primary care doctor has no economic incentive to hold on to the patient and to do his best by the patient from his own resources. Rather than simply underserving the patient, the primary care doctor makes too quick a referral. However much this tendency may prevail in other health systems, it is not a real possibility in the renal disease programme. Since the physician electing capitation payment is already a fully qualified specialist in the renal branch of internal medicine, there is no higher court of appeal to which he can refer his patient even if, on the basis of the fixed price economic logic, he were disposed to do so. Perhaps the essential point, in the wide acceptance of the capitation mode of payment among renal physicians, aside from the critical fact that they are being paid at a handsome rate, is that their medical contribution is distinctly recognised and billed, not being subordinated to, and later extracted out of, a payment to an institution for a total package of services.

Centre Dialysis and Mounting Expense

The early expansion of dialysis during the 1960s and the early 1970s came mainly through home dialysis. It would have been impossible to provide long-term dialysis to thousands of patients, with new cohorts entering every year, through academic medical centres and community hospitals. The Veterans Administration hospitals played a leading role – and still do – in training patients for home dialysis, and for this particular purpose, they have been given an enlarged mandate to serve non-veteran patients. In sequel to the early expansion of home dialysis, and the general optimism about the capacity of many patients to manage dialysis for themselves, it is a striking fact that the proportion of patients on home dialysis has been declining. According to the National Dialysis Registry there were 2,703 home patients in January 1973, and 3,879 such patients in June 1975. However, the 1973 figure represents 37 per cent of the total number of dialysi patients, but the 1975 figure represents only 25 per cent of the total. Two dialysis centres in Washington, D.C. in April 1976 had clinical responsibility for 250 dialysis patients, of whom only 15 were on home dialysis.

Accompanying the decline of home dialysis, there has come a rapid increase in dialysis performed in hospitals and free-standing (non-hospital based), proprietary dialysis centres (also called 'satellite centres', as in the earlier quotation from *Harrison's Principles of Internal Medicine*). In June 1973 there were 500 such facilities, both hospital and non-hospital; by May 1975 there were 747 such facilities (Sub-committee on Oversight of the Committee on Ways and Means, US House of Representatives, *Report,* 22 October 1975, p. 8). Clearly this is a high-growth enterprise, propelled not only by the clinical need, that is, the number of patients in renal failure, but also by the level and structure of federal funding.

Of the 747 facilities existing in May 1975, 606 were hospital-based and 141 were proprietary centres. Most patients are dialysed in centres. However, dialysis technology is diffusing rapidly to community hospitals, though the number of patients dialysed in most hospitals is quite small. In relation to the question of home dialysis versus institutional dialysis, in many hospitals with two or three dialysis machines and the staff to operate them, the diversion of patients to home dialysis would result in an under-utilisation of dialysis equipment and personnel and a significant loss of income to the hospital in relation to its fixed capacities and expenses.

The proprietary centres are single-purpose organisations, designed, equipped and staffed solely in order to dialyse referred patients. Being more specialised than hospitals and also profit oriented, these facilities must dialyse or go out of business. They tend to have a high volume of operation, servicing fifty or more patients, and to be located in metropolitan centres, where the large population produces a threshold aggregate of renal failure patients. Forty such centres are owned and operated by a corporation called National Medical Care.

If the number of referred patients rises rapidly, it is easier to expand the in-house capacity, both staff and equipment, to meet the rising demand or to start a new centre than it is to train and place 'overflow' patients out on home dialysis. Ten years ago, professional dialysis knowhow and dialysis organisational capacity were so critically limited that home dialysis was imperative. Physicians then spoke of the patient's personal motivation, or 'will to live' as being a basic factor in his survival, which had to occur by home dialysis or not at all (Fenton, 1968, p. 1097). What commenced in grim necessity acquired an enthusiastic commitment, so that home dialysis became a socio-medical crusade which prevailed for a time. The patient nowadays is not thrown upon his own adaptive capacity or 'will to live' via home dialysis and can more easily draw upon the substantial long-term assistance of others, through centre dialysis. But, at the level of national policy and fiscal rationality, there is concern that the centre dialysis programme is too expensive. It remains to be seen whether policy concern and legislative incentive can reverse the sweep toward centre dialysis and restore the earlier enthusiastic push toward home dialysis.

To stem the flight away from home dialysis, some physicians, legislators, and public administrators have given serious thought to the establishment of a quota system, or a limit on the number of centre patients. This is a controversial idea because of its potential infringement upon the autonomy of clinical judgement.

In its investigations during 1975, the committee of the House of Representatives which has legislative responsibility for the renal disease programme heard from renal physicians whose practices ranged from a low of 20 per cent of patients on home dialysis to a high of 80 per cent. The physicians who testified were in general agreement that a level of 50 per cent home dialysis is medically feasible (Sub-committee on Oversight of the Committee on Ways and Means, US House of Representatives, *Report,* 22 October 1975, p. 4). Raising home dialysis from the current 25 per cent level to 50 per cent would result in an annual saving of some 21 per cent in the total programme cost. At the 1975 level of programme cost, 21 per cent would amount to $74 million. The renal dialysis programme is certain to expand over the next ten years until an equilibrium is achieved between new patients entering the programme through renal failure and old patients exiting either through death or successful transplantation. The annual dollar savings to be realised could correspondingly rise from $74 million into the $250 million range.

The House Sub-committee using medical arguments about the clinical feasibility of home dialysis endorsed the concept of a quota but its report took note also of dissenting views, for example those of Dr John P. Merrill of Peter Bent Brigham Hospital in Boston. He had led the establishment of home dialysis in the Boston area and published several journal articles which attest to the general feasibility of home dialysis and to its advantages over centre dialysis. His opposition reflects a reluctance to have governmental mandate tip the balance in treatment decisions, as well as an awareness that home dialysis is too difficult an undertaking for many patients. In a letter to the Sub-committee dated 4 September 1975, Dr Merrill stated:

> I am particularly interested in the problems involving home dialysis because of our very early and constant involvement with this modality.
>
> Advocates of home dialysis point to the observed decrease in percentage of dialysis patients being trained for home dialysis as a result of insufficient Federal 'incentives' to home dialysis. In fact, I believe, this began prior to the implementation of Public Law 92-603 and can probably be more closely tied to the availability of alternatives to home dialysis for these patients.
>
> In spite of our early hopes for this procedure as a more convenient and economical form of therapy, it is obvious that there are many patients who exhibit a major disinclination to treat themselves or be treated by spouses or assistants by home dialysis. Many of these individuals are psychologically and emotionally unadaptable to this procedure; others of course are not. I believe that the option for satellite or home dialysis certainly should be given and independence emphasized. However, in my own experience, a good many patients actually feel 'rejected' by their physician if they are urged to undertake home dialysis. It seems to me to be a grave mistake to create in such patients a conflict between more favorable funding

and their own preference. While I am aware that some physicians have been criticized for not attempting to inculcate the desire for home dialysis in some patients, I am equally aware of the fact that group dialysis or satellite dialysis embodies a kind of group psychotherapy which for some mentalities is a much more supportive alternative than is dialysis alone at home.

Thus, I believe strongly that any standard of treatment which is encouraged, fostered or advocated by the Federal Government should have clear-cut therapeutic advantage over available alternatives. A modest and probably debatable economic saving is in my view insufficient reason for the Government to advocate any form of treatment other than optimum. [*Hearings before the Sub-committee on Oversight of Committee on Ways and Means,* US House of Representatives, 24 June–30 July 1975, pp. 145-6.]

No systematic comprehensive studies of socio-economic characteristics of home dialysis patients have been done, but I surmise that the earlier cohorts contained many individuals of high social and intellectual attainment. One listing of thirty patients on home dialysis in 1969 included two lawyers, three physicians and four PhDs (Bailey *et al.,* 1970, p. 1852). The social composition of the first generation of dialysed patients may well have been biased toward upper-middle-class patients who could master the strenuous task of home dialysis. The selective channels by which these early patients in renal failure were referred by community physicians to the first generation of dialysis physicians may have favoured middle-class patients and hindered poor patients. Once in the hands of renal physicians at university medical centres and teaching hospitals, these same patients tended, we suppose, to respond positively to the enthusiasm of the academic physicians for home dialysis, which was in turn an adaptive response to the stringently limited hospital capacity for carrying patients on a long-term basis. With the spread of dialysis technology and organisational know-how to community hospitals, and its extension to 19,000 patients by 1975, dialysis became a broad-scale process conducted in many hospitals and centres, no longer confined to medical vanguard institutions.

Although home dialysis may place a lower claim upon professional resources in the long run, it does require a substantial initial investment in the training of the patient and his or her helper. The training period varies from patient to patient with an average length of two to three months. Following initial periods of experiment and revision, the training process has become systematised at many institutions sponsoring home dialysis, with the development of teaching films, training manuals and courses for training the trainers. However, it still has many irreducibly 'individual' aspects, wherein the patient and his assistant must learn and demonstrate their proficiency at specific tasks, such as monitoring the patient's blood pressure and connecting the blood access point on the patient's body with the dialyser. In its degree of intensiveness, the individual component of dialysis training is quite similar to the skill-learning of medical and nursing students, in learning procedures such as venipuncture and endotracheal insertions.

Many physicians have recently incorporated dialysis into their practice, but part of the lagging emphasis upon home dialysis may be due to the fact that the newer generation of renal physicians is not faced with the necessity of stretching scarce resources, nor of personally acquiring the skills for operating the apparatus. Furthermore, a large complementary cohort of renal dialysis technicians is being trained in the mechanics of dialysis and dialysis machine maintenance. Whereas dialysis training is a relatively minor part of the training of the renal physician, it is the whole of the technician's training. Yet the technician can function only under the supervision of a physician; he has no skills in relating to the patient and it is easiest in an organisational sense for him to perform his tasks in a hospital or dialysis centre. He may be sent out to a patient's home as a competent troubleshooter with the apparatus, but not for general supervision of dialysis.

A patient facing renal failure is not likely to become interested in home dialysis unless his physician has a positive, knowledgeable attitude toward it. Moreover, the physician must be willing to delegate the dialysis task to the patient while maintaining ultimate clinical responsibility himself.

Acquainting the patient with this possibility is, like most communication between doctor and patient, more than sheer imparting of cognitive information. Whatever the doctor says conveys not only its literal content but also the metacommunicative subscript, 'The doctor said it to me.' Simply for the doctor to broach the possibility may be taken by the patient as an injunction. As Dr Merrill's letter suggests, some patients may construe the suggestion of home dialysis as a rejection by the physician. An omission of such mention by the physician may be taken by the patient as an indication of the physician's disapproval or scepticism about this treatment mode.

A further element in the doctor-patient relationship indirectly discourages the resort to home dialysis. The physician who makes the definitive diagnosis of chronic rental failure is likely to be a renal specialist in a metropolitan area. This physician charts the treatment plan and gets the patient set for survival via maintenance dialysis. If the patient enters dialysis at a satellite centre, this same physician will probably retain responsibility for dealing with emergencies, but he is not likely to be routinely involved in on-going dialysis. When the patient enters home dialysis, the patent's 'regular' community physician may serve as the medical resource person, rather than the physician at the dialysis centre, especially if the patient lives far from a dialysis centre. Some home training programmes include a component of training expressly directed to the patient's own physician. The willingness of this physician to educate himself about dialysis and to take clinical responsibility can be an additional limiting factor in the feasibility of home dialysis.

Dialysis Policy and Family Factors

One of the major effects of the federal legislation has been to reduce the amount of home dialysis relative to institutional dialysis and to encourage the growth of free-standing dialysis centres which can service large numbers of patients. Though expensive in absolute dollar outlay, centre dialysis is probably cost-effective in terms of volume of service provided in relation to the input of supplies, equipment and staff labour.

Did the legislative coverage of renal dialysis initiate the trend away from home dialysis or did it merely facilitate and accelerate a change which, reflecting other forces in the socio-medical arena, was already underway? This question arises perennially in the analysis of the effects of planned social innovation, and it is always in principal insoluble. One cannot run an experiment in which one real world unwinds with the introduction of the innovation or policy stimulus, and the other unwinds without it.

Maintenance dialysis began in 1961 with a handful of patients. By 1964, 300 patients were being sustained; by 1972, 7,000; and currently 19,000. The momentum toward the extension of dialysis to more patients was underway before the 1972 Social Security amendment; it also appears that the relative decline of home dialysis was similarly underway, being caused by factors which preceded the legislation, however much the legislation may have accelerated the process.

In my opinion, two factors stand out in accounting for the decline of home dialysis. They are interrelated, and neither is a direct economic factor. The first is the difficulty of fitting home dialysis into the prevailing constellations of family roles. The second factor is the increasing provision of dialysis to elderly patients. A number of investigators have examined the family dynamics of home dialysis, with a particular focus on the husband-wife relationship. I will not review their literature but will make a few remarks based upon their major points of consensus.

Home dialysis was offered by physicians who believed in it, to patients who had an interested and supportive spouse or other family helper. In the early years of home dialysis, the spouse as a rule received more training than the patient. This emphasis accorded well with the concept of the patient as the sick, helpless person in need of care from others. It also accorded with the fact that young and middle-aged renal failure patients are predominantly male. For the wife to minister to the needs of her ill husband, even in a trained capacity, is consistent with cultural conceptions of the wife role. However, the husband was also trained when the patient was female.

At many of the early dialysis units, which were based in academic centres, the emphasis was gradually shifted from training the spouse to training the patient – that is, giving primary training to the patient with a secondary training of the spouse. This change was made on the basis of the independent experience of physicians, social workers and nurses in diverse locations, and their convergent recognition of problems engendered by the original strategy. The primary training of the spouse gave her/him an inordinate degree of initiative, control and responsibility in the dialysis situation; by the same token, it thrust the patient into a role of greater passivity and dependency than the illness dictated. This strategy has been reversed to such an extent that some training programmes now virtually exclude the spouse. The newer concept is: train the patient and let the patient train the spouse (or other household member). Under this concept, the professional trainer makes no presumption about family responsibilities in what is inherently a stressful situation. The partners are free to work out actual arrangements between themselves subsequently in the home. The patient may be trained for completely independent self-dialysis. With a fistula located in the leg, the patient can himself perform all phases of the routine. Yet the presence of an interested, concerned spouse is still deemed invaluable for emotional support if not for concrete assistance.

This account demonstrates the strain which the exacting and time-consuming route of dialysis can place upon the fabric of family interaction. The effort, both emotional and physical, demanded of the patient by home dialysis is greater than the much simpler 'custodial' requirement of centre dialysis. It, therefore, comes as no great surprise that many patients and their families given a choice prefer centre dialysis which requires only that the patient make himself available. Since the centre dialysis patient need not spend his own time in setting up and cleaning the dialysis equipment, he may even have more time for work and other activities than the home dialysis patient.

In keeping with the humane medical ethic of using skill and knowledge to reduce suffering and extend life, dialysis treatment is increasingly offered to patients with infirmities in addition to renal failure. In the first years of dialysis, most selection committees and clinical decision-makers probably followed implicit criteria of social worth. Some imposed a chronological age ceiling, usually at age forty-five or fifty, but they then found themselves making awkward exceptions. As dialysis capacity expanded, less and less was said about chronological ceilings. 'Physiologic age', rather than chronologic age, became the limiting factor. If physicians are reluctant to restrict treatment on criteria of social worth or sheer age, neither are they happy about limiting treatment to 'physiologically worthy' clients.

Older patients are more likely to live alone than younger patients, and, if married, to have spouses who are infirm or disabled. This has obvious implications for the question of home versus centre dialysis. A population of predominantly elderly patients will perforce rely more heavily upon centre dialysis facilities. Figures from the Congressional report show that in 1975 the proportion of sixty-five-year-old and older dialysis patients in relation to the national total was 9.4 per cent (House of Representatives, 24 June 1975, p. 6). However, the proportion was generally much higher in those states such as Massachusetts, Rhode Island, California and Washington, D.C. (which is, of course, not a true state comparable to the fifty 'real' states) with a favourable balance of health manpower and resources in relation to the state's population. This suggests that where the resources are relatively abundant, they will be devoted to the benefit of clients who would not fare as well in less favourably supplied environments. It is a reasonable extrapolation to suppose that, with a gradual geographical improvement of health resources, the proportion of elderly-to-total patients will increase over time.

The mass extension of dialysis includes not only a higher proportion of elderly and infirm patients, but also an increasing proportion of patients who are poorly educated, in marginal economic circumstances, and whose place of residence cannot be adapted to the objective requirements of the dialysis apparatus and process. Renée Fox (1975, p. 709) recently observed:

> . . . in terms of ultimate American beliefs in justice, equality and universalism, it is good that people who are poor as well as those who are rich, people who live in the inner city as well as those from the suburbs and the exurbs, can now have access to these modalities of treatment if they need them. But patients who are economically deprived, who have a minimum of formal education, who do not have intact families, who are dispirited by their unemployment and poverty present a whole array of problems that have implications for their experiences with dialysis.

Dialysing patients with a limited life expectancy (aside from the threat of renal failure), such as the elderly and the patient with other serious illnesses, raises a number of questions from the standpoint of a narrow cost-benefit and rehabilitation rationale. When the spectrum of dialysis patients is expanded to include socially disadvantaged patients, again the question arises of the implications for their treatment. One major implication is that such patients are less likely to be good candidates for dialysis at home. How formidable a barrier 'social disadvantage', in its many aspects, is to a reversal of the trend away from home dialysis remains to be seen. Efforts are underway to formulate more exactly the indications and contraindications for the conduct of dialysis in the home (McDaniel, 1975).

Conclusion

In conclusion, let me briefly restate the ground I have covered. I looked into the background of the federal legislation in the United States for end-stage renal disease and examined its effect in terms of greatly broadening the opportunity for renal failure patients to receive maintenance treatment. A recent *New York Times* article describes the federal legislation as a highly successful experiment which may presage greater governmental support for the treatment of other serious diseases (Anderson, 1976). At the same time, it has been an expensive experiment and it has promoted forms of treatment which are perhaps more costly and less rehabilitative than they need to be. The cost contrast between home dialysis and centre dialysis has attracted particular attention from public policy-makers. The decline of home dialysis and the rise of centre dialysis is perhaps an inevitable concomitant of the more penetrating spread of treatment. The way in which this and other major treatment decisions are made involves a complex set of interactions between the physician and patient, with involvement as well from the patient's family. Economic factors are important, but perhaps no more critical than other factors, such as the extent to which the physician wants to assume on-going clinical responsibility for a patient in home treatment, and the extent to which the patient wants to invest himself in his own treatment. It is difficult, yet essential, in analysing the implications of health policy to keep in mind the major forces which are generated by policy imperatives and, at the same time, to discern the typical attitudes which patients and physicians have toward each other and toward the illness problems which bring them together.

References

Altman, Lawrence K. (1971). 'Artificial Kidney Use Poses Awesome Questions', *New York Times,* 24 October, New York.

Anderson, Alan (1976). 'Dialysis or Death', *New York Times Magazine,* 7 March.

Anonymous Patient. (1976). *NAPHT News,* February, pp. 20-21.

Bailey, George L., Constantine L. Hampers, John P. Merrill and Patricia A. Paine (1970). 'The Artificial Kidney at Home', *Journal of the American Medical Association,* 15 June, 212, no. 11, pp. 1850-55

Beavert, Carolyn Sue (1974). 'Caretakers of the Intermittent Dying: Role Strain of a Hemodialysis Team', Master's Thesis, University of Missouri, May (unpublished).

Burton, Benjamin T. *Kidney Disease Program Analysis – A Report to the Surgeon General,* Public Health Publication no. 1745, US Department of Health, Education and Welfare, July 1967, Washington, D.C.

Congressional Record – US Senate, 30 September 1972, Washington, D.C.

Eady, R.A.J. (1971). 'A Patient's Experience of Over One Thousand Haemodialyses', *Proceedings of the Eighth Conference of the European Dialysis and Transplant Association,* pp. 50-61.

Fenton, Stanley, S.A. Christopher Blagg, Joseph W. Eschbach, Jr. and Belding H. Scribner (1968). 'Treatment of End-Stage Renal Disease by Home Hemodialysis', *Journal of the American Medical Women's Association,* vol. 23, no. 12, December, pp. 1096-103.

Fox, Renée (1975). 'Clinicosociologic Conference – Long Term Dialysis', *American Journal of Medicine,* November, pp. 702-12.

Fox, Renée and Judith Swazey (1974). *The Courage to Fail,* Chicago, University of Chicago Press.

Hallan, Jerome B., Benjamin S.H. Harris III and Albert V. Alhadeff (1968). *The Economic Cost of Kidney Disease,* Public Health Publication no. 1940, US Department of Health, Education and Welfare, August.

Harrison's Principles of Internal Medicine, seventh ed., 1974. New York, McGraw-Hill.

Hearings before the Sub-committee on Oversight of Committee on Ways and Means, US House of Representatives, 24 June-30 July 1975, Washington, D.C.

Institute of Medicine, (1973). 'Disease by Disease Toward National Health Insurance?', National Academy of Sciences, Washington, D.C. June.

LeSourd, David A., Mark E. Fogel and Donald R. Johnston (1968). *Benefit/Cost Analysis of Kidney Disease Programs,* Public Health Service Publication no. 1941, Department of Health, Education and Welfare, August, Washington, D.C.

Lowrie, Edmund, J.M. Lazarus, A. Mocelin, G.L. Bailey, C.L. Hampers, R.E.

Wilson and J.P. Merrill, 'Survival of Patients Undergoing Chronic Hemodialysis and Renal Transplantation', (1973). *New England Journal of Medicine,* vol. 288, no. 17, 26 April, pp. 863-7.

McDaniel, James W. (ed.) (1975). *Proceedings – National Workshop on Rehabilitation and Psycho-social Aspects in End-Stage Renal Disease,* Denver, Colorado, University of Colorado Medical Center.

Roemer, Milton, 'On Paying the Doctor and the Implications of Different Methods', *National Health Care,* edited by Ray H. Elling, Aldine-Atherton, New York, 1972, pp. 118-37.

Strickland, Stephen P. (1972). *Politics, Science, and Dread Disease.* Cambridge, Massachusetts, Harvard University Press.

Style, A. (1976). 'Letter from Mississippi – Life in the Delta', *British Medical Journal,* 17 April, pp. 952-3.

Sub-committee on Health, US House of Representatives, *Background Information on Kidney Disease Benefits Under Medicare,* 24 June 1975, Washington, D.C.

Sub-committee on Oversight of the Committee on Ways and Means, US House of Representatives, *Report,* 22 October 1975, Washington, D.C.

Titmuss, Richard M. (1971). *The Gift Relationship.* New York, Pantheon Books.

Whittingham, Edward (1976). 'A Personal View', *British Medical Journal,* 17 April, p. 955.

It would rarely be denied that traditionally general practice has been accorded a low status within the hierarchy of the medical profession – a dogsbody for the treatment of minor complaints and a gatekeeper to the medical specialisms. More recently, however, especially since the 1960s, the traditional conception of general practice within the hierarchy of the medical profession has begun to disintegrate and to be replaced with the view that general practice deserves the treatment and status 'on par' with any other medical specialism. Subsequently, a great deal of research authored largely by the expanding academia in general practice has been published. Sadly though, sociologists have, to some extent, ignored the relatively virgin field of research into general practice.

Consequently, the following paper by Horobin and McIntosh is welcomed. Not only because it is a report on sociological research into general practice, but also because the research takes an unusual but important theme: the study of the ways in which general practitioners interpret and conceptualise their work and the consequences this has for the ordering of their professional activities. The authors pursue their study by interviewing a number of rural general practitioners to discover how they conceptualise the 'formal responsibilities' of general practice and, in so doing, the paper provides a preliminary description of the conceptual criteria that effect how the practitioners organise their work. Of particular note is the theoretical framework the authors employ in their research. A theoretical framework that places the interpretations and meanings attributed to their work by the subjects under study at the forefront of the analysis and description.

The paper with its interest in the study of the medical profession and its detailed description of general practice, therefore merges neatly into the theme of the volume. However, it also throws a new light into the arena of sociological research into the medical professions and occupations by proposing and demonstrating the use of an alternative sociological model.

C.H.

RESPONSIBILITY IN GENERAL PRACTICE[1]

Gordon Horobin and Jim McIntosh

Introduction

In a review of research in the field of general practice (Royal College of General Practitioners, 1970) the authors noted that 'in order to improve the ways in which we work it is necessary first to know how "work" in general practice is carried out'. The review covered many studies of work in general practice but generalisation was made difficult by problems of definition, and hence of comparison, and by a lack of information on certain aspects of practice, notably variation in work-styles. Richardson *et al.* (1973) found daily consultation rates in 142 practices varying between 31.6 and 7.6 per 1,000 patients and concluded that although variation is 'largely due to the attitudes of patients and this in turn will depend, amongst other factors, on what patients have come to expect of their personal doctor . . . our findings point strongly to the doctor himself as the major source of variation in consulting rates' (p. 141). Other aspects of variation have also been documented, e.g. the use of antibiotics in the treatment of respiratory illness (Howie *et al.* 1971); home visiting patterns (Marsh *et al.* 1972); referrals to outpatient departments (Scott and Gilmore, 1966; Forsyth and Logan, 1968). Research carried out by our colleagues at Aberdeen into abortion, family planning services, male sterilisation and adeno-tonsillectomy has also shown up to ten-fold differences between practices in their hospital referral rates.[2]

Despite the many 'medical' studies, general practice has received rather less attention from sociologists. There are, of course, exceptions, ranging from the general survey perhaps best exemplified by the work of Cartwright (1967) to the detailed study of routines in one practice (Fletcher, 1974). Jefferys and her colleagues have studied 'social problems' in general practice, examined the characteristics of practices in a London borough and more recently, have focused their attention on health centres (Jefferys, 1965; Sidel *et al.* 1972). Mechanic, also using a large sample, has collected useful data on the sources of dissatisfaction amongst general practitioners (Mechanic, 1972). There have also been studies of prescribing (e.g. Dunnell and Cartwright, 1972), practitioners' workloads (Williams, 1970), communication in general practice (Comaroff, 1976) and the consultation process (Stimson and Webb,

1975). In general, both the 'medical' and the sociological studies provide detailed information on more or less specific illnesses or aspects of practice and, simply because they are specific and detailed cannot answer questions about the ways in which GPs organise their work over the whole spectrum of patient-initiated problems. Our concern was not with individual features of general practice. Rather, our emphasis was upon the interpretative and conceptual aspects of the doctor's perceptions of their work as a whole. That is, we were interested in the interplay between GPs' definitions of their role and the total context in which they operated and the way in which this ordered their activities. Variations in specific aspects of GPs' work were therefore to be regarded as indicators of more general variations in work styles. The present paper reports on a modest attempt to approach this topic through a series of interviews with a small sample of mainly rural practitioners.[3]

Orientation

Given this general research task it might appear that our first choice of method should have been direct observation, despite its difficulties. The confidential, private nature of many patient-general practitioner interactions is perhaps the most important of these, although it is not an insuperable one. The observational method is also extremely time-consuming and produces its best results when carried out over a lengthy period of time in, at most, two or three locales. In such circumstances interviews are often used as a poorer substitute or short-cut on the assumption that if you cannot watch what people do, you can, if you are prepared to tolerate an unknown element of distortion, ask them about it. Our reasons for choosing an interview approach, at least initially, were however based on rather different grounds. Our concern was not only with *what* doctors do but also with *why* they do this rather than that. We conceptualised our research question as 'how do general practitioners construct their work from the interplay of the problems presented to them, the context in which they carry out their work and the resources at their disposal?'

The phrase 'how do general practitioners construct their work . . . ?' may require some elaboration. In the course of their everyday life, their interactions with other people and their behaviour in relation to their environment, social actors interpret and give meaning to their social world. This is not to say that all actions are 'thought out'; that would imply a highly rational view of behaviour. It does, however, suggest that all actions, even the most routine and automatic, are subject to interpretation; we attempt to *understand* our own actions and those actions we observe. In this sense each person 'constructs' the social world which he inhabits according to the meanings which he attaches to the objects, actors and actions in that social world. Further, although a number of individuals who share a common culture may construct similar social worlds (i.e. many of their understandings are shared) each construction is unique, based as it is on unique experience.

Work tasks and routines are clearly subject to interpretative action in this way. The more 'routine' the job, the less scope there is for variation in performance, and hence in 'work styles'. 'Professional' work, such as medicine, contains a balance of accepted routine procedures and personal styles. It is variation in such work styles and the meanings attributed to the work that is our primary research interest.

Clearly the ways in which GPs construct their work depend on a variety of 'factors' – their medical training and background, their on-the-job learning in the specific practices in which they have been involved, and the changing ideologies of medicine, illness and health, are some of them. What we have loosely called 'the problems presented to them, the context of their practice and their resources' are themselves interrelated with each other and with the factors already mentioned. Whereas hospital doctors are relatively encapsulated in a 'medical' world – the hospital – GPs are subject to a greater variety of inputs from the non-medical world of their clients, and the other agencies with which they share boundaries – social work, 'welfare', public health, etc. In other words hospital doctors are more free to construct their professional world in professional terms: the GP's world is wider, more permeable to influences from without the medical profession.

The GP typically sees a sample of problems selected according to lay criteria of illness and medicine, whereas the hospital doctor's sample of problems is selected according to professional criteria; the GPs doing a major share of the selecting. Thus a large component of the GP's work, we would suppose, is the initial sorting of problems into various treatment and referral categories – the hospital doctor's work being one of the categories from which he, in turn, does a secondary sort. We further suppose that the categories available to the GP will vary with the context of the practice and his available resources. For example, a single-handed practitioner, remote from hospital and social work services, is in a different context, with different resources from a member of a large urban group practice, and they probably see different samples of problems.

This orientation towards the 'construction of work' suggested the interview as the preferred method of enquiry rather than as a relatively imperfect substitute for observation. Our concerns, in other words, were not primarily with what GPs do, but with how they perceive their job. This focus, in turn, dictated the *form* of the interviews, for, to detect variations in doctors' perceptions of their work, it was important to give the maximum scope for the respondents to choose their own topics and emphases. To legislate for them what were the 'problems' of general practice would, in other words, defeat the object of the enterprise. Needless to say some compromise was necessary since, apart from anything else, an interviewee expects to be asked some questions. Furthermore, we had, from our reading and from discussions with some of our medical colleagues, decided upon several areas of interest which we hypothesised would be relevant to the doctors and would reveal variability between them.[4] Thus, for example, we hypothesised that GPs might face problems in deciding when to refer patients to hospital. Defining and coping with 'trivial illness' and 'social problems' were other topics we tried to cover with all our respondents, although we phrased our questions as generally as possible and only asked them if the topics had not already been covered in the course of our 'interview discussion'.[5] All our interviews were tape recorded.

We decided to interview first a sample of rural GPs, firstly because we assumed (rightly) that they would be comparatively 'under researched' and would be less bound by surgery hours than urban GPs and, secondly, because we wanted to look initially at 'traditional' practice. If general practice is cottage industry compared with the modern industrial enterprise of hospital medicine, then this character should be best typified in single-handed practice in remote areas. Furthermore, simply because most British GPs now practice in urban partnerships or groups, rural practices have been largely neglected.

Most of us live in towns and, for us, easy access to medical care is taken for granted. So we take for granted that we can choose our general practitioner and that, in an emergency, we can be easily admitted to a general hospital containing all the necessary hardware and professional expertise. If we stay in hospital we expect to remain in close contact with our friends and relations. For a significant minority of the British population, however, these assumptions do not hold. These are the people who live in relatively remote, isolated areas. Equally, the doctors and nurses who provide for their primary care cannot assume a readily available set of secondary services. This factor – relative difficulty of access to specialist care – is probably the most important single element in what we have called the context of practice and is hence a primary independent variable in a comparative study of 'constructions of work' in general practice. This was perhaps our major reason for beginning our study in this way; we hoped to trade on our commonsense knowledge of town practice so as to draw out the salient characteristics of practice in isolated areas.

Another important variable which is related to, but not dependent upon, geographical location is the resources at the disposal of the practitioner. In this we include technical aids (X-ray, ECG and laboratory facilities, etc.) and 'complementary' help.[6] Remote practices, in the sense of 'remote from a general hospital', do not necessarily lack such resources. For example, two of our sample of island practices had cottage hospital facilities, and in one of them the distinction between 'general practice work' and 'hospital work' was very blurred. Furthermore these isolated communities tend to have a well-developed district nursing service, with the nurses working closely with the doctors.

In short then, 'remote area practice' is by no means an homogeneous category and some of the variations along these two dimensions, location and resources, will be examined in the rest of this paper.

Analysis

We have chosen the theme of 'responsibility' as both the organising topic and the title of our paper. It is, of course, a theme with many facets and it recurs again and again in the interviews in a variety of contexts. The formal responsibilities of the general practitioner are clear enough. He is responsible for providing primary medical care for his own patients and, in emergencies, for any person not registered with him. If he lacks either the competence or the resources for adequate treatment, he has the responsibility to refer the patient to an appropriate agency, usually a hospital. It is in the practical application of these formal rules that he sometimes faces difficulties and it will become apparent that doctors differ both in their interpretations of the rules and in their application of them. Hence there is variation between doctors in their perceptions and discharge of responsibility.

What sorts of differences are there, then, and how, if at all, are these differences related to the 'objective factors', mentioned above, of location and resources. To simplify this discussion we will concentrate on ten practitioners, five remote from back-up services and five relatively near to specialist facilities. 'Remote' is defined operationally as more than, at a minimum, an hour's journey from the nearest consultant service and more than two hours' journey from a general hospital. Brief details of these practices are attached in Appendix 1.

Conceptualising Responsibility

An important aspect of the doctor's conceptions of responsibility is the notional limits that he draws around his sphere of competence and duty. What sorts of things, in other words, are properly part of general practice and what are not?

Dr 1 Och yes, yes – people sort of come up to talk about their problems and nowadays . . . they may come to a doctor rather than to a minister as in days gone by. This is well known, of course. You get this in towns as well. People will want to talk about marital problems, every kind of problem

JM You don't mind this? It's just part of your job?

Dr 1 No, if I minded that there'd be no point in my being here . . . these things are important to people . . . perhaps one could mention [that] in the country really you are a member of the community, you see. My wife and I take part in quite a lot of sort of community affairs . . .

Dr 13 . . . well what isn't appropriate? This is where I find the advantage of a small practice; one has time . . . You know you have time for this kind of problem and because you are in the community, you know just who to phone up.

Dr 21 When you talk about responsibility I feel pretty strongly about it because I think it is a duty. I feel that if I have a patient it is my duty to see that patient right as far as possible and that is irrespective of what it is.

GH Do you think it is part of general practice? A proper part of general practice giving advice and listening to social problems?

Dr 21 I think somebody has to. I think it is part of the things we should do because there is nobody around available to do it . . . if you get somebody who was miserable and fed-up and about to put their head in the gas oven and through a combination of support and helping them through the crisis and rearranging their life situation, you in fact make them happier people, this is very rewarding and probably makes it worthwhile in the end.

Dr 14 . . . what is a little more difficult sometimes is to be able to sort of refer this to perhaps the new paramedical supports, new ones are growing up like your social workers and welfare people and all this sort of thing.

JM Why is that?

Dr 14 Well I think it is because you are accustomed to dealing with it yourself and often, I don't know, I quite enjoy sometimes doing this sort of sorting things out with people and, I don't know, I think we can still sometimes get a little quicker action say from a government department than perhaps a social worker can get you see . . .

JM Would you say that non-medical problems are ever inappropriate to general practice?

Dr 14 Oh no, I think this is very much part of my job . . . but you see you are stuck in a place like A——— where one knows all that is going on. One knows the people, one knows to some extent what their financial situation is, you know their boats are doing well, you know they are having a bad time, you know if they are on the verge of bankruptcy or whatever, you know if somebody is drinking too much. There is not an awful lot that goes on over any length of time in a town this size that you don't get to hear of it, so that you are generally aware of the context of the patient's problem before the patient explains it to you . . .

Dr 16, in contast with the above, while he did deal with the multiplicity of non-medical problems with which his patients presented, would have ideally defined his role more narrowly.

Dr 16 You see to me a doctor is a scientist. He should try his best to be a scientist all through. Only then can he do justice to his profession. However sympathetic or kind one wants to be towards a family he can't be a social worker. If I am a social worker I am doing an injustice to my profession; there are a lot of problems that could be easily isolated from general practice making me a real doctor or scientist . . .

This topic is obviously associated with the doctors' relationships with social work. Until fairly recently, social work was very under developed in the Highlands and Islands and the GPs had little choice but to be interested in 'social problems'. Since regional reorganisation, however, the number of social workers in these areas has increased and some doctors resent the intrusion of the profession upon their traditional preserve. Part of the reason for the demarcation dispute lies in a failure to understand what social workers 'are supposed to do', with the result that 'problem cases' come back to the GP, apparently unsolved. There appear to be no such problems in the doctor-nurse relationship, presumably because district nurses tend to work from the general practice, especially in the remoter areas. Interprofessional relationships and courtesies are apparently better understood between the two older professions, but lead frequently to friction between these two and the social workers.

The breadth of the doctors' professional role, as indicated by their attitudes towards 'social problems', is also closely related to their perceived place in the community. As in the above quotation from Dr 1 the topic of non-medical problems leads 'naturally' to one of community involvement, itself a many faceted phenomenon. For some doctors, being part of the community is one of the more satisfying aspects of practice in such settings.

JM Could I ask you what you would say were the main satisfactions in practice in this sort of area?

Dr 13 Well, for me, I think quite honestly it is being part of the community. This is something that has grown and, as I said, I would hate to leave B———. I now feel that this is my home, this is where I belong and I am part of it. I don't know whether people agree with that in B——— but this is how I feel . . . Friends do your work, you know this feeling of being part of what is a real community.

Dr 20 When you've been here some time you get to know most of the people and I sort of hope they treat me as a friend and you look in on them and chat about the weather and fishing and the crofting thing and you know you get more . . . that's why I like it, a country practice. [But] it can be infuriating because I think they take advantage of you to some extent . . .

However, such involvement in the community is double-edged. From one point of view it can mean being unable to quarrel with patients who are also neighbours.

Dr 9 This is a flaw in me . . . I have to *like* my patients too.

GH Are there some you don't like?

Dr 9 Oh yes, there are some I don't like. I bet there are some who don't like me . . . It's very rarely that people here openly quarrel with their neighbours; although they may hate them, it never comes up to the surface and the same thing with me . . . in fact I would say that I've never had a quarrel but there must be some dislike me intensely, think I'm a rotten doctor and they've to put up with me, and I with them . . .

Dr 13 You can't quarrel with people in a small community like this where everybody is related to everyone else and if you quarrel with Joe Bloggs you suddenly discover about fifty people will be related to them and another thirty went to school with them.

It can also make it very difficult to form close relationships.

Dr 21 Well of course the worst thing you can have is a friend who is a patient . . . it can be very embarrassing. If you know a lady very well you don't very well want to do internal examinations. Therefore I think so far as possible you don't want to make a patient a friend or a friend of a patient. In a country area it is very difficult to avoid doing this, so in fact you just sort of shut your eyes and charge on and pretend they are not friends. Otherwise you would not be doing your job properly. It is difficult to take up small talk after in fact you have been in a, shall we say, an intimate, compromising sort of situation like that with your patient.

Dr 1 The closer you are to a person, the less easy it is to treat them properly [but] unless you're a hermit, you see, it's difficult to remain completely detached. Neither Dr R nor I ever go and drink in the pub . . . we have our friends certainly but at the same time we have to be very careful.

So this embeddedness in the community has rewards and problems. You cannot, as the community's first resort in times of trouble, ignore the family relationships of your patient, treating him purely as a 'medical problem'. The more you involve yourself in the lives of your patients the more diagnostic leverage you can exert and the more you can anticipate problems. But this involvement means that you can never really be off duty. Patients cannot hide from the doctor and the doctor can never hide from the patients. Thus, 'knowing' the patients and the community in this involved manner has important implications for the doctor's style of work. As an example of this we may consider the decision to refer to a hospital. There are, of course, different kinds of referral: for diagnosis, confirmation of diagnosis, advice or treatment; emergency, urgent or 'cold' treatment. All the remote doctors experience occasional difficulties in emergency or urgent cases, although they differ in the degree to which they regard referral *per se* as problematic.

Dr 1 We have no hospital in this area. We have a very good hospital in C———— and we have very good hospitals in D————. To go to C———— you have to cross the water in the ferry and to go to D———— involves eighty miles of travelling so that you really have to consider very carefully, you know, whether you're going to send a patient into hospital . . . we do tend to treat ourselves more serious injuries and illnesses . . . and people here do tend to trust us a lot more . . . and don't demand to go into hospital every time something serious happens.

Dr 9 It's a worry I have and have had ever since I graduated, how much you should send to hospital . . . I hope I don't oversend, but of course if I tried to make sure that there's something badly wrong before you chase them off to hospital you're bound to make the odd mistake . . . if you do make a mistake, it's a real bloomer . . . should I just say 'send them [maternity cases] off a fortnight before, and what do I care if Dr 11's beds are full up, what do I care if she's leaving seven kids behind with only her husband to look after them?' Now, should I say that or should I hang on to them and maybe have to deliver her myself, if something else goes wrong? Am I wrong? These are the things that worry me at two o'clock in the morning when I can't sleep.

Dr 13 . . . you look very carefully before you send them thirty miles for an X-ray . . . one day somebody is going to have a massive haematemesis and then being thirty miles is going to be a nightmare. But then you could be ten miles away and stuck in a traffic jam I suppose, this kind of thing. I always think very carefully about sending a coronary in . . . I would really hate to send a coronary and have it die on the way.

However, if distance from back-up facilities were the only, or even the most crucial factor in determining attitudes towards referral, we would expect that the greatest difficulties would be experienced by those doctors who were most remote from such facilities and that for those with relatively easy access to support systems it would be relatively unproblematic. But, while this proposition was in general supported by the data, it was by no means always the case. For example,

Dr 10 does not appear to be especially concerned about problems of referral despite his physical isolation.

> Dr 10 One treats quite a lot and . . . we've a reasonable laboratory service at D———— they are extremely good and we get a quick return, so we can carry out most of our investigations before we refer . . . a lot of [referrals] are for treatment and of course occasionally one is stuck oneself, but again, of course, general practice is like this, I mean, you've got to channel the patient into the right department in the hospital . . .

On the other hand, for another doctor with much easier access to a hospital, decisions about whether or not to refer appeared to constitute a major problem.

> Dr 16 . . . I came to this part, as a matter of fact to be honest with you I didn't know whether they had a hospital near by. Lots of times I am in a dilemma. It is very difficult to make up your mind whether a child has a broken leg or not. You have to send them for an X-ray. The nearest place is E———— – thirty-eight miles from here, which is ridiculous. Here, forty miles is not a small distance . . . There are lots of circumstances where you need a consulting unit near by . . . I had a young girl, eighteen years old; she comes with a cut on her forehead . . . she was absolutely pale. So I brought her in, cleaned her up and gave her a cup of coffee and put in a couple of stitches. Now, a dilemma. All my findings, external examinations, gave no evidence of internal damage. I am convinced but still I am not justified in keeping her here, I should send her to a consulting unit . . . There are lots of circumstances where you have to take a decision. If you err on the right side you are playing safe, if you err on the wrong side, just once, you regret life-long . . .

This was probably in large part a product of the expectations with which he entered his present practice, these expectations in turn being based upon his experience of the availability of resources in another rural context in which he had previously practised.

> Dr 16 The impression that I had was that there would be some hospitals around, and I didn't bother to find out more about it because I came from (an English County). Its population is about 250,000 and they had an enormous amount of facilities. F————

city there is a hospital and another eight miles there is another hospital, ten miles there is another hospital, twenty-five miles G———— hospital. All round there are hospitals. That was the impression I had that there would be at least some hospitals.

It seems then that it is the *perceived,* rather than the objective distance from services which is important in structuring practitioners' attitudes towards referral.

Whilst all doctors take into account a variety of factors in deciding whether or not to refer they differ apparently in the *range* of non-clinical factors and in the *weight* they give to them. This is again partly related to distance from hospital in that a long journey can be seen as both a health risk (e.g. myocardial infarctions) and as a psychologically depressing influence on the patient and patient's family (e.g. for elderly people, hospital is where you are sent to die, isolated from home and family). Now we would argue that the more deeply involved the doctor is with the lives of his patients the more problematic is the decision to refer when the clinical pay-off from hospitalisation is possibly marginal. At one extreme the decision, probably taken in consultation with next of kin, is whether or not to let the old person die at home.

Dr 19 [Trainees have got to learn that] sometimes it's kinder to let an old person die at home than to get a diagnosis. They don't want to go to hospital. You find that some old people, you know, that you send them to hospital, they may get first-class treatment but they'll die in a week; they'll be unhappy, whereas if they die at home . . .

Dr 9 But you're asking what my worries, my problems. This is the sort of thing that worries me, when to send patients. You get an old lady of eighty with carcinoma of the breast – do you send her off to Glasgow? Well maybe if they amputated her breast she'll live to be eighty-five; if they don't amputate her breast, if I don't send her away, maybe she's going to die in six months. Now my feeling is not to send them off, but am I wrong, and how the devil can you tell? Do you send her away and before they've amputated her breast she's so terrified of being in hospital that she just ups and dies and I've had that happen. I find I promised them specifically that they wouldn't die and I'm damned if they didn't.

Differential perceptions of the relative costs and benefits of hospitalisation will of course produce different patterns of treatment. Some remote area doctors keep coronary cases at home, others keep 'old hearts' at home and send away 'young hearts'. Again these differences are related to objective distance from hospital but this, by itself, does not explain the differences.

We have suggested that the definition of the GPs role can be fairly elastic, spreading into virtually any area of human or 'social' problems. But even within the area of the 'purely medical' (itself, of course, a flexible concept) there are differences. Their perceptions of the oft-quoted 'problem of trivial illness' is illuminating. Without exception our respondents saw the treatment of trivial illness as a necessary, albeit sometimes irritating, part of general practice, for, as one GP pointed out, almost all illness is minor at some stage. They all agreed that discriminating between the trivial and the serious was a necessary part of their job as a GP.

> Dr 13 How can you discourage? They have got to come to you before you can decide that it is trivial . . .

There was also, of course, the very practical concern that what seems to be trivial may turn out not to be.

> Dr 13 There are some where we see them so often with trivia that you reach the stage where you examine them obsessionally because one day they are really going to have something wrong with them and, that's the day you'll miss it. You are terrified you'll miss it and you probably encourage the vicious circle . . . I go to see her, and I get summoned at all sorts of odd hours. She can't get her breath, she is being sick or something. The last time she couldn't get her breath and when I went there I walked in just as she was lighting a cigarette. And yet I feel I have to go. Every time I'm summoned I have to go. One day she might have an obstruction or she might be . . . and this is very time-consuming. It is very difficult for me.

Further, while the complaint itself might be classified as trivial, part of the GP's job is to alleviate patients' fears and hence these calls on their time are seen as legitimate.

> Dr 14 You get called out sometimes at a ridiculous time to a ridiculous complaint. But when you visit the patient you realise that they don't think it's ridiculous and its worrying them and, you

know, your annoyance melts – at least, I hope it does.

Those doctors who have had previous experience in larger urban practices say that they are much less troubled by trivia in the country. This is sometimes explained as being due to a more stoical and considerate attitude on the part of rural patients. 'Our patients are very considerate here' was a very common sentiment. Dr 10 ascribes it to a closer doctor-patient relationship:

> in a group or partnership the patient says 'Well there's somebody there, that's what they're there for' morning, noon and night . . . whereas [here] they do realise that if you're on your own that you're on twenty-four hours of the day, and they've got much more respect for you.

Dr 1 sees certification as the key to the difference:

> There's more demand for medical certificates down South; there's far more pressure put on patients by the employers. Whereas here, you see, the nature of the work is totally different, many of them are fishing or working for themselves . . . so they may not come to you . . .

but he goes on: 'and down in the South, too, people on the whole tend to be less considerate'.

One category of patients tend, however, to produce more trivia and, in a sense, they become, for the rural GP, the equivalent of the city GPs 'malingerers and time-wasters'. These are the temporary residents, the summer visitors.

> Dr 9 Visitors in summer are just a bloody nuisance. Somewhere between 50 per cent and 75 per cent of the time, they shouldn't be going near a doctor at all.

> Dr 20 I mean midge bites, for instance, we get people coming in with midge bites or sunburn and you wonder why on earth they ever come . . . but you've got to appreciate that it worries them . . . my wife got a phone call from the hotel with a woman saying her sister was shaking all over. So my wife said 'What's the trouble?' and she said 'Oh, she put salt on her grapefruit instead of sugar, and she's taken a mouthful', and could I come at once . . . Sheer panic.

There may sometimes, as some doctors recognise, be good reasons for panic.

> Dr 19 There's no proper accommodation for them, they're sleeping in a tent, and they've had a minor accident or got soaked, exposure. You can't get them to bed . . . You can't really ask a bed and breakfast place to take them in, you can't put them in a first-class hotel . . . they've maybe got hundreds of miles to travel home.

'Trivial illness', we would argue, is not so much a category of illness as a product of pressure of time and inadequate resources. It may, however, be significant that the visitors are singled out for opprobrium for they constitute precisely that category of patients who feel no responsibility towards the doctor and for whom the doctor in turn can have no long-term responsibility. Nor, not knowing the patients and their histories, can he afford to dismiss their claims to his attention if only for fear of subsequent litigation should 'things go wrong'.

In treating patients who attend the surgery or who call him out, the doctor has no choice but to diagnose and treat whatever 'medical problem' is presented. But does he have a responsibility to do more than that? Can he and should he take on an entrepreneurial function rather than just serve in the NHS cateteria?

The practitioners in our sample agreed that, while patients have the right to medical care when they ask for it, they also have the right to refuse medical care when they do not want it. But clearly preventive medicine depends upon doctors taking the initiative in at least making health care (as opposed to 'illness care') available. General practitioners are understandably somewhat chary of preventive work since they have usually neither the time nor the resources for more than fairly straightforward screening. So as far as the treatment of illness is concerned, the patients themselves *normally* have to take the initiative. Yet doctors do act on a relative's say-so when the patient is a child, an old person, or 'in an emergency'. The rule is, then, that if a patient is physically able to call upon the doctor and does not do so, even under pressure from relatives, then the doctor must respect his right to avoid treatment. There are difficulties in adhering to such a rule though.

> GH I mean, how far can you go worming out the truth from somebody. For example, a patient consults you about an illness, I mean, does that imply then you've got responsibility to get to the bottom of it, regardless of the patient's privacy?

Dr 15 Undoubtedly yes. After all in the first instance the patients have joined our list voluntarily, they have chosen us as their doctors, they've put themselves in our care. If they come with a complaint it's up to us to get to the bottom of it and put it right, whatever this entails. Very often of course they don't come and present the full facts to you, you've often got to drag an awful lot of it out and it is not unusual for one to be painfully aware that you're not being told the truth. Some of them must honestly think we're charlies the things they expect us to believe. I would use any method which I thought was appropriate to find out the truth.

GH I suppose there must come a point, I mean, when the patient says 'look I'm not going to tell you about that, that's my affair'.

Dr 15 Well I would very promptly say then 'I'm sorry, there's no point in me wasting your time and you wasting my time, I cannot help you. You've come here with a specific complaint, as far as I'm concerned the history is relevant to the alleviation of your trouble and if you're not prepared to tell me, then it's pointless going any further.'

Dr 21 I tend to be an interventionist so that I might perhaps go out of my way to visit their wife or perhaps even try to waylay them and say to them 'Look you are not looking well, are you feeling all right?' It is very difficult and it doesn't often happen actually. If they were a danger to themselves or a danger to somebody else you would obviously have to intervene. I don't think it is at all pleasant charging into a situation when in fact you are not wanted and, as I say, if somebody wants to die of TB or cancer of the lung without medical attention I think they are entitled to do so.

So, for the most part, practice in these remoter areas involves a conception of responsibility which is perhaps both wider and deeper than that which is usually held to characterise general practice. Until fairly recently general practice appeared to be the Cinderella of the NHS, relegated in some discussions to a role which is little more than that of a 'referral agency'. That formulation of the role of primary medical care has, we believe, been superseded by one embodying a more strategic place in the reorganised health service, partly because of the renewed emphasis, in a time of economic recession, on 'community care'. At the same time, the health centre movement seems to have been predicated on the assumption that GPs wish and should be encouraged to function rather like hospital specialists, albeit on a less exalted level. In such practices, GPs would specialise along their own lines of interest in e.g. paediatrics, geriatrics, etc., do more diagnostic work with the readier access to technical aids and refer more easily when appropriate to cognate professions such as social work. But more traditional forms of general practice persist even in cities, though they are understandably more in evidence in rural areas.

To conclude our presentation and discussion of the data, then, we return to some more of those aspects of responsibility which provide both the problems and the satisfactions of rural practice. Single-handed practices are especially demanding in that the responsibility is undiluted and continuous, but the doctors welcomed the opportunities they had for exercising their clinical expertise autonomously.

> Dr 10 I was beginning to find when I was in [the city practice] that it was becoming less satisfying, that with the hospital next door and the, sort of, patient mentality, everything had to be treated at hospital. Since I've been up here it's become very satisfying again because I can really practise medicine again.

But being in solo practice produces a good deal of strain.

> Dr 9 I can't even take my boat very far off shore without making sure that somebody can see me, see where I am, and give a shout or send out a boat after me.

> Dr 16 . . . I am at it all the time. Tuesday is my half-day which means I am not consulting in the evening. Sometimes I go to E————. Every hour I ring back to see what is happening in the village.

One aspect of this heightened responsibility can often be an inability to switch off.

> Dr 7 I've never been able to switch off completely from – what is it? guilt? I've lost many a night's sleep. I should be thankful, I'm sure, that I didn't make more mistakes . . . We are very fallible people, GPs, and I think medicine as a whole is like that. If you have learned the lessons of medicine, it should keep you pretty humble.

On the other hand:

Dr 21 Normally I have a very good shut off and I never lose a minute's sleep over worrying about a case. I make my decision and that is it and I tend to stick with it.

Occasionally, remote practice can even be exciting!

Dr 10 . . . and Dr R's got one very isolated spot, a five mile walk across the hills, or the way we usually go is by boat. I've only once been called out there myself on his day off and unfortunately we never got there. We were cast adrift from the fishing boat in our small boat in a force 8 gale. There was a reception committee waiting for us but they waved us off; they realised that we were going to be smashed to bits if we tried to land on the rocks. We made two attempts and then gave it up and eventually got picked up by the fishing boat half way down Loch H————. We had to chase after it because every time he hoved to to try to get a line out to us he started drifting into the rocks. It was quite an adventure.

GH It's just as well you don't get too many of these calls.

Dr 10 Yes. As far as I'm concerned this all adds interest to the job.

There are also occasional veterinary jobs:

Dr 19 . . . we had a trainee who was a registrar in anaesthetics . . . and one of the local people brought up her dog with a fish hook in his mouth and [the trainee] happened to have a consultant anaesthetist staying with him. So they both came up and they tried to anaesthetise the dog and failed, so in the end we had to use brutal methods . . . [the hook broke] and they were annoyed at being beaten by this dog and wanted to persevere. But I said no – the time had come to admit you're not as good as someone else – you have to turn a patient down and in this case it was a dog.

and unexpected hazards:

Dr 19 . . . and if there is any real problem you can often ring up [a consultant] and get advice over the phone. Especially now – you couldn't so much in the past because we had a manual exchange, but now we've an automatic exchange and we can talk in privacy – before, we couldn't.

Of course our isolated doctors were self-selected – they chose that kind of practice for many individual reasons: boredom and frustration with the 'daily grind' or urban practice, dislike of city life, desire to be on one's own or simply a feeling of kinship with people and place. With very few exceptions then, any disadvantages are clearly outweighed by the satisfactions – of home life:

Dr 1 My wife got absolutely fed up with life down in L———. My daughter hardly knew me. Now, you see, although I work fairly hard, and maybe work long hours, I do have time at home to see my wife and children – they know who I am . . .

. . . and of the job itself:

Dr 10 I enjoy it, I enjoy people . . .

Dr 9 You must have confidence and you must show you have confidence. You come to a house where something awful is happening and they're all in a terrible state, you know. Now I suppose this is just appealing to my sense of power, being able to walk in and take charge and in a minute or two they are settled down and they are not panicking because you've arrived and all their burdens are on your shoulders. This I find profoundly satisfying as long as I can, in fact, cope with what's happening. By this I don't mean that I can cure the patient necessarily but I can cope with the situation . . . It's not much fun being a GP nowadays . . . but if it's fun anywhere, it's fun out here. I admit with shame, I've delivered an extended breech with the nurse giving chloroform at one end, and praying, and me delivering at the other end, and swearing, and the baby lived, and the mother was all right. Now when you've done that, it's almost like winning the pools. I shouldn't ever have got myself into that situation . . .

Conclusions

We began this discussion by asking how perceptions of general practice might be related to geographical location, especially relative remoteness from hospital facilities, and available resources. While all the doctors who are located at some distance from hospital recognise that this fact places extra responsibility upon them, they orient to it in rather different ways. They do not all feel that remoteness is the dominant characteristic of their work situation. On the other hand one, at least, of the relatively 'near' doctors (Dr 16) feels extremely isolated. Again while being single-handed obviously deprives some of the relaxation of time off, this does not appear radically to differentiate their perceived work styles from those who are in partnership.

On the other hand, in providing their accounts of their practices, the doctors do appeal to the perceived constraints of their individual practices; i.e. common formulations of their responses were: '*here* you have to do . . . '; 'in this *practice,* I have to'; '*it's different here*'; or, less commonly, '*in practices like this*'. General practitioners seem very aware of possible differences in work-styles and in their orientation to various aspects of their work, and they attempt to explain such differences at least partly by invoking a certain uniqueness in the conditions under which they work. In other words they tend not to say, 'I *choose* to do this' but rather, 'of course, *here one has to do this*'.

And of course there *are* unique features of each practice; 'remoteness' is so general a characteristic as to be virtually meaningless. Dr 10 is remote in terms of sheer distance from hospitals but he can make time-off arrangements with another single-handed doctor. Dr 1 and his partner are remote but they can have fairly ready access to a small hospital, as can Dr 9 albeit with rather more transport difficulties. And so on. But in addition each doctor brings to his practice an orientation to work based partly on his previous practice experience. Drs 1 and 10 both came to their present practices from very overloaded urban practices and consequently find comparatively few problems. Dr 16 had of course previously practised in a rural area which was much better served by back-up facilities. Finding his expectations unfulfilled, he accordingly identified problems of isolation and referral as being of major importance. Amongst the doctors from whom we have not directly quoted, Drs 11 and 12 combine general practice with medical and surgical work respectively in their 'own' small hospital, and Dr 36 grew up in and eventually took over a practice which his father had run for almost half a century and consequently faces the problem of 're-training' his patients. All these elements of individual biography clearly influence the doctors' views of general practice, but, within the quite broad limits set by biography, by physical location and by the agreed canons of good clinical procedure, the doctors have a good deal of freedom in constructing a viable work role. Given all this, we were more surprised by the similarities in their accounts than by their differences.

Some time ago we prepared a discussion paper based on these data under the title 'Rationalising General Practice'. We used the term 'rationalising' to indicate the quality of interview data. We came to regard the things the doctors told us not as more or less adequate descriptions of what they did, but rather as attempts jointly with us (the interviewers) *to make reasonable* (rationalise) General Practice as a job. As in any interview, we were forcing our respondents to pay attention to and talk about aspects of their lives which, however important they may be, are seldom verbalised. In this sense they are, in what they say, 'constructing' the work of general practice out of the material available to them; unassembled 'facts' about things they have done, fugitive ideas about their work – its tedium, irritations, satisfactions, etc. – their perceptions of what general practice may mean to others, their interpretations of what we wanted, etc. In these interviews, that is, we – interviewers and interviewees – 'conspire' to produce accounts of general practice which 'make sense' in the context of the conversation.

But does this mean that we cannot say anything about the nature of general practice from our interview data? We would expect that the accounts provided by the GPs would almost certainly have been different if we had asked different questions, the same questions in a different order or in different forms, or even on different days. Repeated interviews or, better still, interviews combined with observation, will perhaps enable us to say more about how these GPs construct their work. Without such 'triangulation' we are forced to be tentative in our conclusions. But we are not purists. We believe that the accounts we have elicited in these interviews can stand as approximations – 'hypotheses' if you like – to be confirmed or falsified if or when further data become available. Clearly we can have greater confidence in some parts of the interview material than in others. Presumably further interviews or observations would not significantly alter their answers to the questions 'How many patients do you have?' and 'How is your practice organised?' These 'facts' are the more or less fully formed bricks which form the foundation of their constructions of work. At the other extreme are their responses to questions which have, for them, an essentially hypothetical character, referring to feelings, ideas, ambiguities, etc., which are not perhaps oriented-to features of work.

A modest 'validation exercise' was carried out. Earlier in the research we fed back a 'working paper' to our respondents, inviting critical comment. Most of the comments suggested additional topics rather than criticism of the points we did make. These additional topics included: financial problems; effects on prescribing behaviour of advertising, drug salesmen etc.; the problems for the isolated doctor in keeping up to date; the ethics of industrial action; and social responsibility to the community. Most thought our account was 'fair, though incomplete' and none expressed any great surprise. A few decided that any attempt at generalisation would be bound to fail – 'GPs are such individualists'. We agree.

We have also reinterviewed some of the doctors a year later and in one case carried on a 'running interview' for a week while accompanying the doctor on his house calls. We are also collecting some data on surgery consultations, home visits, referrals and cottage hospital in-patients. Whilst adding new data, these have not thrown any real doubt on the 'validity' of the original interview material: the accounts remain 'reasonable'.

In the end then we have to stick our necks out and say 'we think this is how general practice *is* for these doctors', although we have not by any means reached that stage yet. The task we have set outselves is, in short, such that we have to use the interviews as a resource; to treat them only as topics for analysis might be an interesting enterprise and one we should like to pursue. But it is not, for us, the primary objective of our study.

Notes

1. A version of this paper was prepared for the BSA annual conference, Manchester 1976, but, because both authors were ill at the time, was never formally presented. We apologise to those who missed the opportunity to discuss or challenge our work but are grateful to those who have given us their comments.
2. We gratefully acknowledge the help of our colleagues especially Drs Barbara Thompson and Mick Bloor in making their data available to us.
3. Our long-term intention is to study variations in work-styles across a range of practice types – urban/rural, large groups, small partnerships, single-handed practices, etc. – by a variety of research methods including observation. This paper is based on the first phase of this enterprise, interviews with about forty GPs, half of them in rural practice. We hope to discuss differences between urban and rural practices in a subsequent paper.
4. We would like to thank Professor Ian Richardson and his colleagues in the Department of General Practice at the University of Aberdeen for the very considerable help and advice they gave us, especially in the early stages of our research.
5. 'Interview-discussion' is perhaps a more appropriate term than 'interview'. The discussion element was apparently recognised by our respondents as several of them used the term or equivalents such as 'talking things over' in subsequent contacts.
6. Although doctors tend to use the term 'ancillary' we prefer to avoid it because of its literal connotation of subservience. Whether or not the doctors treat such help as subservient is a separate empirical question.

References

Bloor, M.J. (1976). 'Bishop Berkeley and the adenotonsillectomy enigma', *Sociology*, vol. 10, no. 1, January, 43-61.

Cartwright, A. (1967). *Patients and their Doctors.* London, Routledge and Kegan Paul.

Comaroff, J. (1976). 'Communicating information about non-fatal illness: the strategies of a group of general practitioners', *The Sociological Review*, vol. 24, no. 2, p. 269.

Dunnell, K. and A. Cartwright. (1972). *Medicine Takers, Prescribers and Hoarders.* London, Routledge and Kegan Paul.

Fletcher, C. (1974). *Beneath the Surface: An Account of Three Styles of Sociological Research*. London, Routledge and Kegan Paul.

Forsyth, G. and R.F.L. Logan. (1968). *Gateway or Dividing Line?* London, OUP.

Howie, J.G.R., I.M. Richardson, G. Gill and D. Durno. (1971). 'Respiratory illness and antibiotic use in general practice', *J of Royal College of General Practitioners*, vol. 21, pp. 657-63.

Jefferys, M. (1965). *An Anatomy of Social Welfare Services.* London, Michael Joseph.

Marsh, G.N. R.A. McNay and J. Whenell. (1972). 'Survey of home visiting by general practitioners in North-East England', *BMJ*, vol. 1, pp. 487-92, 19 February 1972.

Mechanic, D. (1972). *Public Expectations and Health Care.* New York, John Wiley & Sons.

Richardson, I.M., J.G.R. Howie, D. Durno, G. Gill and I. Dingwall-Fordyce. (1973). 'A study of general practitioner consultations in North-East Scotland'. *Journal of the Royal College of General Practitioners,* vol. 23, pp. 132-42.

Royal College of General Practitioners (1970), Present State and Future Needs of General Practice (Report No. XIII).

Scott, R. and M. Gilmore (1966). 'The Edinburgh Hospitals' in *Problems and Progress in Medical Care,* ed. G. McLachlan, London, OUP for NPHT.

Sidel, V.W. M. Jefferys and P.J. Mansfield. (1972). 'General practice in the London Borough of Camden', *Journal of the Royal College of General Practitioners,* supplement no. 3, vol. 22.

Stimson, G. and B. Webb. (1975). *Going to See the Doctor,* London, Routledge and Kegan Paul.

Williams, W.O. (1970). A Study of General Practitioners' Workload in South Wales 1965-1966. Reports from General Practice No. 12 London: Royal College of GPs.

Appendix 1

Dr 1 Has 1 partner. 2 district nurses. 2,000+ patients plus large temporary resident population. 80 miles from district hospital. 10 miles + ferry to nearest small hospital. 11 years in general practice, 8 in his present one.

Dr 9 Single-handed. 20 years in rural practice, 11 of those in his present one. 2 district nurses and 1 health visitor. 22 miles by sea from nearest cottage hospital and 120 miles by air from general hospital. 1,300 patients + sizeable casual summer trade.

Dr 10 Single-handed. 27 years in general practice. 3 years in present practice –

800 patients. Previously in a mixed urban-rural single-handed practice with 3,500 patients in the South. 2 district nurses. 57 miles from an 80 bed hospital over fairly poor roads. A further 90 miles by air from there to the general hospital.

Dr 13 Single-handed. 1,200 patients. 1 nurse attached. 6 years in general practice. 30 miles from general hospital.

Dr 14 In general practice for 30 years all of that time in his present practice, a 6-man group with 13,000+ patients. 1 full-time practice nurse, 2 district nurses, 3 health visitors. 35 miles from general hospital.

Dr 15 Has 1 partner and 4,000 patients. A general practitioner for 25 years, 23 of those in present practice. 2 part-time district nurses and 1 health visitor. 16 miles from hospital.

Dr 16 Single-handed. 7 years in general practice, 1 year in present practice. 1 district nurse. 1,100 patients. 38 miles from hospital.

Drs 19 & 20 A two-man partnership, 1,600 registered patients which can swell with summer visitors to 4,000-5,000. Dr 19 has been 4 years in the practice, Dr 20 has been there for 8 years. The nearest consultant hospital is 65 miles away.

Dr 21 Single-handed. 23 years a general practitioner, 14 in present practice. Practised previously in an urban area. 2,300 patients. 2 district nurses and 1 health visitor. 17 miles from hospital.

Medicine, like other professions, has long been male dominated. This is not a new or recently uncovered feature of professional groups, but a bias which is tacitly acknowledged in research and then ignored in preference for studies on social class, status or socialisation. Fortunately, Elston ignores social class for sexism, and thus it is the sexist division of labour which forms the central theme of her paper. Through a careful historical analysis, she illuminates the strategies by which male supremacy is built up and maintained within the medical profession.

Elston rightly focuses on two key areas of control – through entry into the profession, and through subsequent career prospects. She first offers an account of selection procedures to medical school. Challenging the accepted explanation of an erratic but steadily increasing intake of women into medicine, Elston argues instead that women have always been treated as a potential resource, allowed into the profession in increased numbers largely when market demands require extra personnel – during the two World Wars, for example, or today when dependence upon immigrant doctors to fill non-career posts becomes politically and economically less viable.

Once trained, it is often argued, women fail to make full use of their medical education. In career terms women are less successful, accepting positions in low status specialities or part-time employment and often leaving work for childbearing during the crucial stage of postgraduate training. Elston again tackles traditional sociological explanation on the grounds that they have failed to reveal both the lack of career choice open to women, and the underlying assumption that it should be the woman who has to combine home with career. A more fruitful interpretation would be to see such continuing discrimination as a further form of occupational control, in this case one which serves to relieve men of competion for the more prestigious hospital appointments.

Sadly, Elston's paper only briefly considers current changes outside medicine which will in time have some impact on the expectations and demands of women doctors. Within medicine, present solutions continue to bend employment possibilities for women round her accepted role of wife and mother, by offering ways in which she can acceptably combine training and work with her domestic role.

It is notable that the sexist bias in medicine is not without its reflection in sociological work. Not only has this aspect of professionalism been generally studied by women researchers, but at a theoretical level, discussion of occupational control has typically ignored one major area of intra-professional conflict, that of the domination of one sex over another. By highlighting the various strategies by which such domination is achieved, Elston usefully brings into focus an important aspect of the process of professionalisation.

M.E.R.

WOMEN IN THE MEDICAL PROFESSION: WHOSE PROBLEM?

Mary Ann Elston

Introduction[1]

The proportion of women entering medical school in Britain is now almost 40 per cent, and among practising doctors almost 20 per cent. Within medicine the increase in the number of women doctors is accompanied by increasing concern with the 'problem of women doctors' (e.g. *BMJ*, 10 January 1976, p. 56). This problem is expressed at two levels; first, in terms of the problem for the community that women doctors pose because of their 'wastage' of expensive training; and secondly in terms of the difficulties faced by individual women doctors in reconciling the conflicting demands of work and family, factors which are often seen as the sole cause of 'wastage'. However, to perceive the employment of women doctors as necessarily problematic in these terms is to ignore the way the changing structure of the medical labour market shapes both female and male medical careers. In particular it fails to account for the way the staffing structure of the National Health Service, especially in the hospital sector, has been predicated on 'wastage' of doctors.

The use of different conceptual frameworks in the analysis of men's and women's working patterns obscures the fact that the latter are, at least in part, dependent on labour market demand and the former on family commitments. The use of the 'life-cycle' and family situation as the sole independent variable relating to women doctor's working can be a legitimation of discrimination rather than an explanation of 'failure' (see Smith, 1976). There are a large number of surveys of British women doctors almost all of which present static pictures of employment patterns related to such factors as marital status, parity and age of children in terms of women's dual careers (e.g. Aird and Silver, 1971; Flynn and Gardner, 1969; Jefferys and Elliott, 1966). The inadequacies of sociological explanations of women's employment in terms of women's dual roles have been cogently criticised (e.g. Barker and Allen, 1976a; Beechey, 1976, Wolff, forthcoming 1977) and the arguments are equally applicable to women in medicine.

Consideration of the position of women in medicine highlights the lacunae in contemporary arguments. Doctors have been regarded almost universally as a white male middle-class group, an assumption justified in the empirical situation for almost a century following the 1858 Medical Act, but not in the current situation where one fifth of practising doctors are women and one fifth are from the Indian subcontinent (Community Relations Commission, 1976). The importance of these taken-for-granted characteristics of doctors as a basis for the power of the medical profession has been neglected. This is in part because of uncritical acceptance of analyses of the American situation where women doctors have until recently been almost invisible (see Lorber, 1975). More importantly, it is because theories of professions and professionalisation, notably Freidson (1970) and Parsons (1951), have continued to emphasise professional-client relations, while neglecting the processes by which occupational control may be exercised by a dominant social group. Such control is exerted not only over the lay public and would-be competitors (see Parry and Parry, 1976), but also over members of the profession, notably junior doctors, women and ethnic minorities (see Elston, forthcoming).

Analysis of the historical and current situation of women doctors must involve a discussion of the factors that have structured the demand for medical staff and also a consideration of why and how it is that women are to be found in certain sectors.[2] This paper represents a first attempt to do this using the, admittedly limited, available data to look at the history of women in medical schools and at the history of employment patterns in the twentieth century.

Women's Entry to Medicine

A widely accepted explanation of the history of women in the professions and specifically in medicine in Britain since 1900 is that of the 'S-shaped curve,' a sequence of 'breakthrough to acceptance followed by stagnation' (Oakley, 1974, p. 79).

> Between the Census years 1921 and 1931 in the decade immediately following the first opening of the doors to women in many professions, the number of women in higher professional work in Britain rose nearly twice as fast as the number of men, by 3% a year as against 0.8%. This was the classic decade of breakthrough. From 1931 to 1951 the two rates of growth were much closer together, (women 3.6% men 3%). But from 1951 to 1961 the number of men went on growing at 4.5% a year while the number of women actually fell by nearly 1% a year . . . This actual fall in women's share in

> higher professions did not continue throughout the first half of the 1960s but neither did women resume their advance (Fogarty *et al.*, 1971, p. 21).

This 'S-shaped curve' has been often interpreted as either due to women's failure to live up to the standards set by the early pioneers, i.e. their motivation is at fault, or to some kind of inherent logic of women's professional development, an autonomous process unrelated to the social conditions in which the development occurs. In the case of the medical profession at least this account needs considerable elaboration to be even descriptively adequate and is in no sense explanatory.

It is not clear exactly what these 'rates of growth' imply. To speak of percentages when the absolute number of women is so small presents a misleading picture. Taking census data gathered at ten or even twenty year intervals and converting them to a per annum basis results in rates unrelated to political and economic conditions and obscures the fact that numbers entering medical school can vary considerably from year to year, as can 'labour wastage'. Because there was no census in 1941 the impression is given of there being no effect from the Second World War on women's activity in the professions, an impression which we know to be mistaken.

Apart from the unsatisfactory statistics, the 'breakthrough, acceptance, stagnation' sequence is open to more fundamental criticism. It implies there are social processes underlying these statistics but no evidence apart from the statistics themselves is produced. The number of women in any profession is a function of the number qualified to practise and the number of those qualified who do practise. The history of medical school selection shows that till very recently there have been strict controls on women's entry to the profession. Women's 'opportunities' to practise have varied since 1921 not because of differing degrees of acceptance but because of changes in the medical labour market.

Fogarty *et al.*, locate the First World War as the time of 'opening of doors'[3] to women in the professions. That the war should bring about a significant numerical increase in the number of women medical students illustrates the inadequacies of the 'dual career' approach in explaining women's activity in medicine, and the need to look at the demand for medical staff. In 1910 approximately 2 per cent of qualified medical practitioners in Britain were women, but by 1921 this had risen to 7 per cent of practitoners and 10 per cent of students in training. During the war the demand for doctors was such as to enable the London School of Medicine for Women to double its intake, with a consequent demand for more beds for clinical instruction than the Royal Free Hospital could provide. Eight of the hitherto exclusively male London medical schools agreed to admit women clinical students as a wartime measure only.

Immediately after the First World War, as after the Second, there was concern about oversupply of doctors and the pool of applicants and entrants contracted. The number of places available for women fell as the male London schools withdrew their clinical facilities for women. By 1925, only University College offered twelve places a year to women (on stricter terms than men), and this situation remained almost unchanged until after the Second World War. By 1938 the London schools were training 40 per cent of all doctors, so that their virtual exclusion of women students was a significant factor in accounting for the low proportion of women students overall. In 1938, 6 per cent of London medical students, excluding the School for Women were women, compared with 20 per cent in the Scottish and provincial universities (Goodenough, 1944, p. 98). London medical schools were not totally financially linked with the University of London until the Second World War. Between the wars, they were heavily dependent on attracting sufficient students and the revolutionary step of admitting women was seen as a deterrent to men.[4] Between 1921 and 1939 the proportion of women students entering medical school rose only from 10 per cent to 15 per cent. The greater growth rate for women doctors in the decade 1921 to 1931 was not a 'breakthrough', but the result of the significant but temporary disruption of the First World War, Fogarty and the Rapoports, by choosing an inappropriate starting point have interpreted a temporary fluctuation as an indication of an underlying trend.

During the Second World War there was an increase in intake by some provincial medical schools but not on the scale of 1914-18. Possible reasons for this may relate to the lower military casualities and hence lower demand for armed forces medical staff. The major effort was in the creation of the Emergency Medical Service hospitals at home for the casualties that never materialised. In contrast to the First World War when women doctors treated casualties at the battle front, in the 1939-45 war they were excluded from the RAMC (Bell, 1953). At the end of the war 25 per cent of medical students were women, and this proportion was not exceeded until 1968. There were falls to around 20 per cent of entry immediately after the war, with 90 per cent of places reserved until 1949 for ex-service entrants, and between 1956 and

1960, in response to the Willink Report recommendations (see below).

The war period saw two significant developments, the negotiations over the proposed National Health Service and the move to financial support from the University Grants Committee by the independent London medical schools. In 1944 the Report of the Interdepartmental Committee on Medical Schools (Goodenough, 1944), set up to determine what kind of medical education would be appropriate to a National Health Service, declared that no barriers other than aptitude should operate in the selection of students. It proposed that coeducation should be the norm in all schools including the ten London schools which, at that time, were single sex institutions (and thus the London School of Medicine for Women should also admit men). In order to bring about this state of affairs Goodenough recommended 'for Government decision that the payment to any medical school of Exchequer grants in aid of medical education should be conditional upon the school being coeducational and admitting a reasonable proportion of women students' (op. cit., para. 5.8, p. 99). Their idea of a reasonable proportion was one fifth. 'Otherwise the women will not form a sufficiently numerous body to ensure a proper status and position. The grudging admission of a few women is unsatisfactory . . . There must be no sense of inferiority or of privilege' (op. cit., p. 99).

In the event the minimum quota laid down by the UGC was 15 per cent, which was the pre-war national average proportion in medical schools. There remained major differences between schools, and the impact of the Goodenough Report in terms of numbers was not great. The medical profession's reaction to the Report appears to have been somewhat grudging. For example, in the Report of Medical Curriculum Committee of the BMA entitled *The Training of a Doctor*, published in 1948 as a reply to Goodenough, we find, 'the conditions under which Government grants are now given to medical schools ensure *no unfair* discrimination against the admission of women students, though here the potentialities of marriage and *consequent loss to the community* cannot wholly be ignored in assessing the ratio of men's to women's admissions' (op. cit., p. 13, italics added).

The post-war medical school selection policies have been in part subject to the quasi-egalitarian ideology of the state (Holter, 1971) culminating in the recommendation to abolish the quota system entirely, issued by the Committee of Vice-Chancellors and Principals in 1973, and the 1975 Sex Discrimination Act. Specific selection and education policies were left, however, in the hands of the medical schools, and the General Medical Council. The Parrys (op. cit.) have described the strategies of social closure adopted by the medical profession (with regard to entry to the profession) to achieve and maintain their high status since the nineteenth century. Over the last thirty years selection in medical schools is claimed to have become more 'objective', in that it is increasingly based on examination performance rather than on social background. Thus medicine, like other occupational and educational fields, shows the shift from 'collectivist' to 'individualistic' rules of exclusion, the latter taking the form of 'credentialism' (Parkin, 1974, p. 6). Such a move is justified on the ground that it selects the 'best' students, but as Parkin points out the relationship between individual capacity and educational performance is distorted along class lines, and selection by examination results alone has not led to a significant increase in the proportion of working-class medical students (see for example Todd, 1968).[5] However, because of the 'weeding out process' in women's education (see Shaw, 1976) the qualifications of women applicants tend to be higher. Some form of covert discrimination therefore became necessary to prevent the number of women rising too much. Thus while the Goodenough Report established quotas 'officially to let women in' they subsequently became weapons for keeping women out, or at least to limit their numbers.[6] The 'separate but equal' treatment of applications for medical school up till 1974 enabled medical schools to claim that there was no discrimination, in so far as the same proportion of female applicants as of male were accepted. Recently, as quotas are being abolished, very slightly more female applicants than male are tending to be accepted. Thus in October 1964 women formed 28 per cent of applicants for medicine and 24 per cent of accepted students, rising in 1969 to 26 per cent applicants, and 27 per cent admissions and in 1974 30 per cent applicants, and 34 per cent admissions (UCCA, 1975). Jefferys, Gauvain and Guleson in 1965 and the Royal Commission on Medical Education (Todd Report) in 1968 found that there were large variations between different schools in their acceptance of women. Excluding the Royal Free (50 per cent women) in 1965 the London Hospital had 11 per cent female students and Leeds 35 per cent. The proportion of women admitted appears to be related to the pressure of applicants per place. The process of weeding-out all but the best girls through the influences of home and school cannot explain the large differences found in 'A' level grades between male and female entrants. As quotas have, to some extent, been abolished women have formed an increasing proportion of medical students while, simultaneously, the standard of 'A' level grades among male entrants has also risen.[7]

The number of places for medical students is related to the estimated need for medical staff, as was clearly shown by the Willink and Todd Reports (1957 and 1968, respectively).[8] Overall medical staffing levels and the distribution of posts by grade and sector are the outcome of negotiations between the leaders of the medical profession, concerned to protect their position, and the health service administration, concerned to contain costs (Elston, forthcoming 1977). Women are scarcely represented on the policy-making bodies of the profession. In 1975, forty-two of the forty-six members of the General Medical Council were men, as were forty-eight of the fifty doctors on the BMAs Council (see Bewley and Bewley, 1975).

In 1975, out of 359 chairs in the London medical schools twelve and one deanship were held by women. In the rest of the country in the same year only two women occupied chairs. (These chairs were predominantly in the less prestigious pre- or para-clinical fields.) Women doctors as a group have little power to influence decisions that affect their employment prospects, notably in the alteration of educational requirements to serve staffing needs.

Women Doctors and Wastage

For most of its existence the National Health Service has had to 'struggle with two unbalanced equations' (*BMJ*, 3 January 1976, p. 3). First, annual medical school output in Britain (currently 3,000) has exceeded the number required to replace the retiring or dying doctors in career posts, predominantly consultants and general practitioners (estimated at 2,500 for 1976), but has been less than the new numbers that are required to staff hospitals at junior levels (4,500 in 1976). The second imbalance is the simultaneous oversupply of would-be entrants to certain fields and shortages in others. As suggested above, responsibility for the structure of the medical labour market lies at least partly with the profession's leadership, among which women doctors are scarcely represented. Thus the National Health Service inherited a 'competitive apprenticeship' staffing structure in the hospitals: the consultant leading a team of junior doctors simultaneously being trained and providing routine medical care. Immediately after the war this pyramidal structure appeared extremely unbalanced with large numbers of demobilised doctors employed as supernumerary registrars. Expansion of the consultant grade was resisted particularly on grounds of cost and the subsequent battles over dismissal of the excess junior doctors have been described elsewhere (Eckstein, 1960).

The significance of these events for 'women doctors' is two-fold.

First, the situation in the fifties is a clear example of the way the structure of the medical labour market in hospitals (and, because hospitals are the major employers, in the health service as a whole) is predicated on 'wastage': junior doctors 'fall off the career ladder' into general practice, into emigration or out of medicine altogether. Second, an analysis of the specific historical situation gives some indication of why it might be that the proportion of women active in medicine remained almost constant at 16 per cent to 17 per cent between 1951 and 1961. The oversupply of doctors led to intense competition in Britain for jobs of all sorts and the belief at least that emigration significantly increased. Not only is it likely that many women doctors will have been unable to find jobs, because of a preference for male candidates as 'better risks' and more 'deserving of employment', but there was also no reason to create posts 'suitable for women' to solve staffing problems as has subsequently been the case.

The ideology of full-time motherhood (and the associated paradoxical elevation of domestic responsibilities to non-work that is both obligatory and essential) has frequently been linked with the post-war withdrawal of women from paid employment. To speak of post-war withdrawal is to take a very short-term view; rather, in medicine as in other fields many women were temporarily conscripted or encouraged into wartime employment. The work of Bowlby (1952) and others is often blamed for the return of women to full-time housework and motherhood but such academic research neither develops in a social vacuum nor is in itself a force for social change. However, it is at least possible that women doctors (and their predominantly doctor husbands) through their formal training and professional socialisation have been particularly exposed to the thesis that full-time maternal care of young infants is necessary for *healthy* child development. What is good for patients' children is good for doctors' children. As Bell (1975) has pointed out, the language that women use to describe the home responsibilities that affect their employment is not one of choice. Women doctors have been frequently criticised for 'preferring' motherhood to the fulfilling of their responsibilities to the community that has paid for their training. However, if a woman accepts that motherhood is her prime responsibility and if there are no alternative child-care provisions it is not a question of 'preference'. Moreover, if a woman believes that her working outside the home may result in maladjusted children, then to do so may be seen as irresponsible to the community.

The apparent excess of doctors in the early fifties led to a fall in medical school intake even before the 10 per cent cut back in places recommended by the Willink Report in 1957. By 1960 this cutback had been reversed as expansion of the hospital sector brought increased demand for 'pairs of hands', particularly to staff the peripheral hospitals and 'unpopular specialties'. Expansion of the consultant establishment and the creation of a permanent sub-consultant grade has often been resisted by the leaders of the profession, e.g. the British Medical Association. The alternatives are to expand the junior 'training grades' and to rely on 'wastage' to relieve the consequent career blockage, or to expand temporary and/or part-time posts which are not on the career 'ladder'. The past twenty years have seen the adoption of the first solution generally and specifically in the use of doctors from overseas seeking further training. Overseas doctors appear to be considerably over-represented in the lower grades and less popular specialties (see Community Relations Commission, 1976).

Concern over the drying up of the supply from overseas, in part induced by the profession's own manipulation of the registration requirements, has led to the call for expansion in the output of British. medical schools. The Todd Report called for a doubling of the 1968 intake by 1990 to alleviate the problem of dependence on overseas doctors (op. cit., 1968, p. 24). Their targets and timetable for expansion of medical schools were not accepted officially.[9]

The second and more recent solution to the demand for 'junior' staff has been the expansion of non-career posts and part-time opportunities. The growth of the latter is usually explained as a function of demographic changes, freeing women of domestic responsibilities leading to the increased pressure from women for part-time posts. Part of this increase is indeed due to the introduction of special part-time training schemes for women doctors (see DHSS, 1969) discussed below, but these schemes would not have been introduced had they not been seen as necessary to solve certain staffing problems. For example, a *British Medical Journal* leader discussing the position of women doctors was quite explicit about the need for 'extra pairs of hands': 'One of the Service's unsolved problems is the disparity between the numbers of training posts needed in the hospital service and the numbers needed to staff the junior grades. Part of the solution could come from more and better use of the pool of medical women willing to work part-time' (*BMJ*, 10 January 1976, p. 56).[10]

So, the pattern of medical staffing under the NHS has seen an increasing distinction between service and training posts in hospital medicine; in this way the medical labour market increasingly resembles a dual labour market as described by Barron and Norris (1976). They suggest that labour markets can be dichotomised into primary and secondary sectors such that,

1. There is a more or less pronounced division into higher paying and lower paying sectors.
2. Mobility across the boundary of these sectors is restricted.
3. Higher paying jobs are linked into promotional or career ladders, while lower paid jobs offer few opportunities for vertical movement.
4. Higher paying jobs are relatively stable, while lower paid jobs are unstable (op. cit., p. 49).[11]

Secondary market posts are likely to be occupied by holders with specific social characteristics, such as minority race or sex. The characteristics of such posts become conflated over time with the characteristics of their holders. The over-representation of women and overseas doctors in lowgrade posts and unpopular specialities has frequently been noted. However, labour market demands alone cannot explain why it is women who tend to fill secondary grade posts, as illustrated in Tables 1, 2 and 3, and unpopular specialties.

Table 1 Hospital Medical Staff†: Analysis by Grade and Sex (England)

	1963			1970			1974		
	Total No.	F	%F	Total No.	F	%F	Total No.	F	%F
Consultant	7,132	412	5.8	9,229	669	7.2	10,603	894	8.4
Senior Registrar	1.090	123	11.3	1,608	218	13.6	2,105	338	16.1
Registrar	3,456	496	14.4	4,362	655	15.0	4,472	773	17.3
SHO	2,693	430	16.0	4,709	895	19.0	6,782	1,348	19.9
HO Pre-Registration	1,613	369	22.9	1,846	414	22.4	2,046	541	26.4
SHMOs & Medical Assistants	1,603	289	18.0	1,218	342	28.1	1.165	381	32.7
Para 94 Appts*	3,258	536	16.5	4,988	1,066	21.4	6,066	1,461	24.1

Source: DHSS 1976 *Health & Personal Social Source Statistics, 1975.*

†Table excludes Junior Hospital Medical Officers, House Officer post registration and others.

*This refers to those staff to whom paragraph 94 of Terms and Conditions of Service of Medical and Dental Staff apply, mainly those carrying out part-time hospital appointments, i.e. clinical assistants.

Table 2 General Medical Practitioners (England): Analysis by Age and Sex

	1965			1968			1974		
	Total No.	F	%F	Total No.	F	%F	Total No.	F	%F
All ages	20,195	2,067	10.2	20,115	2,306	11.5	21,531	2,975	13.8
30-35	2,230	238	10.7	2,190	288	13.2	2,323	411	17.7
Unrestricted Principals				18,731	1,831	9.8	20,219	2,526	12.5

Source: DHSS, 1976, *Health and Personal Social Service Statistics 1975*

Table 3 Local Authority Medical Staff (England) (NB: these figures are whole-time equivalents)

	1969			1973		
	W.T.E.	F.W.T.E.	%F	W.T.E.	F.W.T.E.	%F
All Grades*	2,212.5	1,113.9	50.3	2,331.9	1,266	54.3
MOH	319.8	12.4	3.9	308.9	17.1	5.5
Deputy Division MOH	246.1	43.8	17.8	220.3	61.4	27.9
MOs in Senior Posts	386.6	237.3	61.4	558.5	356.3	63.8
MOs in Departments	1,045.3	727.7	69.6	987.9	704.1	71.3

Source: DHSS Statistics and Research Division
*'All grades' includes other staff not mentioned below.

Table 1 shows how the increase of women hospital doctors has taken place primarily in the lower level posts and in the non-training grades (i.e. the grades where the greatest overall increase has occurred).[12] Table 2 shows that women doctors form an increasing proportion of general practitioners especially in the young age group, but are under-represented as unrestricted principals. Table 3 shows that while women formed over 50 per cent of the old Local Authority Medical Staff they were concentrated in the clinical medical officer grades. While statistics concerning the non-consultant grades in the reorganised community medicine sector (a low-status branch itself) are not yet available, of the

559 consultants in community medicine posts in 1975 119 were held by women (21 per cent).

The explanation of the concentration of women doctors in particular sectors of medicine must involve consideration of their position in society as a whole, and the sexual division of labour in the family, a division seldom questioned by those who complain of women doctors' wastage. Davies (1975) quotes an anonymous medical administrator giving evidence to the Select Committee on the Anti-Discrimination Bill: 'If we train one hundred men, then in five or ten years' time we shall have one hundred doctors in full-time practice; if we train one hundred women then we shall have only thirty per cent working in five or ten years, and then most probably in part-time work' (op. cit., p. 132). This statement is not only a total misrepresentation of available evidence on working patterns of both male and female graduates, but also highlights the ideological assumptions behind the concepts of 'quotas' and 'wastage'. The question which needs to be asked is: 'What counts as wastage and to whom does it represent loss?'

There are numerous studies of women doctors' wastage but very few of men's. From past patterns it would appear that after ten years, of Davies' hundred men, at least one will be dead or have given up practice and fifteen will be in practice permanently outside the United Kingdom. A number of studies have shown male doctors are more likely to emigrate than women. Bewley and Bewley (1975) also point out men are more likely to die or become incapacitated through illness and more likely to be struck off the Medical Register. Most surveys in the sixties showed that at any one time 35 to 40 per cent of women doctors under the age of sixty-five were working full-time, and another 35 to 40 per cent part-time (e.g. Flynn and Gardner, 1969; Aird and Silver, 1971; Jefferys and Elliott, 1966; Whitfield, 1969).[13] A survey of Aberdeen graduates ten years after qualifying showed that one third of graduates of both sexes were not contributing to British medical manpower (Ogston, Dawson and McAndrew, 1969).

Further, to speak of wastage implies that the activities of those married women doctors who are not in full-time work are of less value than (available) alternatives, and also implies that men and women have equal non-work commitments. The assumption that it is women who have primary responsibility for childcare and home maintenance is seldom questioned in medicine. This domestic labour is seen as non-work and the cost to society of replacing it is ignored.

The work of women who do practise may be regarded as wastage because of its undemanding nature; it is suggested 'married women need not be condemned to a soul-destroying routine of contraceptive clinics' (*BMJ*, 10 January 1976, p. 56). The leader does not ask who will staff contraceptive clinics if women doctors do not.[14] It does put forward the idea that women, because of their inevitable family commitments, must resign themselves to being excluded from the 'demanding branches of medicine' for if modifications in training in these fields were introduced 'standards would inevitably fall'. Analysis of the horizontal distribution of women doctors suggests that several branches of medicine are dependent on this underutilisation (in terms of both the nature of the work and hours).

The concept of 'demanding specialties' conflicting with family commitments and its converse, of certain specialties being particularly suitable for women, assumes that the division of labour in the family is inviolate, an argument which obscures the historical structure of the medical labour market. Within hospital medicine specialties differ in power (in terms of resource allocation) and prestige and in terms of financial reward, as exemplified by the distribution of Distinction Awards and the opportunities for private practice (see Elston, op.cit.). Until very recently hospital medicine (at consultant level) in terms of power, prestige and financial rewards, ranked above general practice and community medicine below both. Table 4 shows that women doctors are unevenly distributed across specialties at all levels, and the same is true of overseas doctors (CRC, 1976). Women are well represented in anaesthetics, paediatrics, child psychiatry and radiology and recently there has been an increase in female consultants in obstetrics and gynaecology. With the exception of the latter, 'women's specialties' are 'shortage' specialties in which the number of posts available exceeds the supply, and opportunities for private practice are limited. Women are under-represented in the surgical sector in which most specialties are 'oversubscribed', and consequently the provision for part-time training is very restricted.[15] These are the so-called 'demanding' specialties, in which 'total commitment' is called for.

A widely accepted explanation of the concentration of women in certain fields is that of reduction of role conflict by women, e.g. 'Women doctors tend to manage their professional career by selecting for work those fields of medicine and that type of practice which are least likely to offer work duties incompatible with the female task' (Kosa and Coker, 1965, p. 295-6). This approach suggests that women will choose specialties (a) in which they have special expertise or experience because of their primary roles as women, wives and mothers or (b) which have suitable working arrangements to fit those primary

Table 4 Women Doctors as a Percentage of the Total by Grade and Selected Specialties, England and Wales (30.9.74)

	Consultants	Senior Registrars	Registrar
All Specialties:	8.3	15.6	16.9
Surgical Group*	1.6	1.6	3.0
General Surgery	0.9	0.6	3.0
Trau & Ortho Surgery	0.9	none	0.2
Urology	none	none	none
Plastic Surgery	1.3	none	none
ENT	4.0	6.0	3.0
Medical Group*	6.5	10.3	13.3
Paediatrics	15.5	26.8	30.9
General Medicine	2.9	4.7	9.0
Geriatrics	8.1	8.2	12.5
Rheumatology & Rehabilitation	10.4	14.3	17.9
Opthalmology	4.1	6.3	9.2
Obstetrics & Gynaecology	12.2	12.6	24.1
Pathology	10.0	28.6	38.7
Anaesthetics	15.8	27.1	31.0
Radiology/Radiotherapy	8.9	17.1	23.1
Mental Handicap	16.7	31.6	21.1
Mental Illness	8.5	21.7	25.2
Mental Illness (Children)	30.7	44.6	60.0

Source: derived from tables in DHSS 1976 *Health & Personal Social Service Statistics 1975*
*includes more specialties than those listed

roles. What the central 'female task' is, and that women are free to choose their field of work and their level of activity is taken for granted by Kosa and Coker. They do not consider that working arrangements, conditions and definitions of what is relevant experience are not immutable and are socially constructed. They fail to distinguish between characteristics of posts and characteristics of occupants, and take the structure of the medical labour market as an historical constant. They,therefore, cannot explain why some apparently unsuitable specialities are chosen and some apparently suitable ones are not (Epstein, 1971; Lorber, 1975). Obstetrics and gynaecology above all fulfil the criterion of special expertise, but, until very recently, there were few women consultant obstetricians. The unsuitable working conditions prevailing in obstetrics and gynaecology, i.e. emergency and night work, are not only frequently used as an argument against it being suitable for women, but are seen as so intrinsic to the specialty that part-time training is not acceptable. Dermatology, ENT, opthalmology and plastic surgery would all seem to be fields where women's special knowledge is as great as men's and working conditions ideal, yet women are not strongly represented.

The community health services (including family planning) have often been regarded as the ideal career for female medical graduates in the same way as teaching has been for women graduates in general. Kelsall *et al.*, point out that for teachers this has been something of a mixed blessing, in that the relatively ideal working conditions and plentiful vacancies (until recently) has resulted in, 'comparatively little pressure for substitute care arrangements or for comparable working arrangements in other types of employment . . . it has actually served to dampen the demands of highly educated women for changes' (op. cit., p. 153). However, it is arguable that rather than community medicine being the ideal field for the female medical graduate, married women have been the ideal labour supply for community medicine when there is a shortage. Because of their other commitments, and lack of other opportunities they have provided a cheap and flexible labour pool in under-financed fields.

Another area where women are, contrary to stereotype, over-represented at the lower levels is in academic medicine, or rather in the basic medical sciences (see Blackstone and Fulton, 1973 and 1975). In recent years medical schools have found it extremely difficult to staff pre-clinical departments with medically qualified personnel because the salary levels are considerably below clinical levels. The result has been increasing employment of non-medically qualified personnel and, secondarily, women. However, they form a small proportion of academic staff in clinical subjects.

Solutions to the Problem? Part-time Training

It has been suggested above that there have been increases in the opportunities for women to work in medicine, particularly part-time, but that these opportunities have not necessarily increased chances for women to have careers in medicine equivalent to those of men. For this to happen more fundamental changes in women's position, not just in medicine, but in society as a whole, are necessary. This would begin to break the circle in which women's position in the family both restricts and is used to justify the restriction of participation in the labour force.

As it is, two solutions to the 'problems of the professional woman's career' are normally proposed: the part-time pattern, and the discontinuous pattern of a break while children are young. The Merrison Report, for example, assumes that part-time activity is the necessary and sufficient solution to women's problems. '*Lastly*, we mention a point which is particularly important to the use of the skills of women doctors. This is that the arrangements for accreditation and thus specialist registration should be flexible enough to allow training on a part-time basis' (Merrison, 1975, para. 142, p. 43, italics added).

The reasons why part-time or discontinuous working is not satisfactory for women wishing to pursue professional careers on a level with men have frequently been noted. They are just as applicable to medicine as other careers (see Blackstone and Fulton, 1975, Lopate, 1968). To qualify for promotion it is essential to keep up with the latest work and to develop and maintain colleague and sponsor ties. This is hard for women to achieve if they work part-time or have a break in the continuity of their employment at a vital stage soon after graduation (when women are most likely to have to take a break). From the feminist point of view it also perpetuates the unsatisfactory situation 'whereby women are disproportionately liable to work part-time, for reasons such as undemocratic family structure and inadequate public provision of child-care facilities' (Blackstone and Fulton, op. cit., p. 271).

The attitude to 'part-time' work in medicine is ambiguous. When done by women it is often seen as failure to utilise fully their state-provided training. For the consultant, on the other hand, it may be the hallmark of success enabling him (or occasionally her) partially to opt out of the state-funded service. Ironically, as Fogarty *et al.,* (op. cit., p. 27) point out, the scope for flexibility in hours and delegating often increase when one is at the top of a career. Women who work part-time at an early stage and, more especially, those who stop work altogether at an early stage in their careers are unlikely ever to reach the top. Only a few women can arrange to cope without some break from full-time work at childbirth under present conditions. The problem is when to time this break. From the career point of view it is better left till late so that a career is well established, but women doctors may be influenced by their training to take account of the increased risks incurred by delaying childbirth.

The Department of Health and Social Security has adopted the part-time solution in the form of special training schemes for married women.[16] The most recent is the Retainer Scheme whereby women doctors are paid £75 per annum to cover registration, medical defence fees, journal subscriptions and work at least twelve paid sessions a year. Table 5 shows the uptake of the scheme with considerable variation between regions. Some 300 women doctors out of an estimated

Table 5 Doctors Retainer Scheme Status Report: March 1973–September 1975

RHA	March 1973	Sept. 1973	March 1974	Sept. 1974	March 1975	Sept. 1975
Northern	10	18	19	18	18	19
Yorkshire	10	9	10	11	14	15
Trent	4	10	6	7	8	11
E. Anglian	6	9	11	11	14	13
N West Thames	24	33	33	18	21	20
N East Thames	9	13	14	11	7	9
S East Thames	14	17	18	19	19	19
S West Thames	17	19	14	16	18	16
Wessex	10	10	11	12	12	12
Oxford	9	12	15	17	17	12
S Western	16	25	22	17	23	26
W Midlands	10	10	9	10	15	17
Mersey	–	–	4	4	2	2
N Western	19	21	17	15	18	17
Totals	158	206	203	186	206	208

Source: DHSS Statistics and Research Division

2,000–2,500 eligible have entered the scheme. More significant has been the provision for supernumerary part-time training posts and the splitting of posts under HM (69)6 (DHSS, 1969 and 1976). It is this measure that accounts for a significant proportion of the increase in part-time posts described earlier. However, as suggested above, the reasons for the implementation of such a scheme at that particular time may be in the demand for doctors in certain specialties. These posts are training posts and there is no guarantee that consultant posts will be available. Like the Retainer Scheme the implementation of the scheme varies from region to region and is dependent on the enthusiasm of particular individuals (post-graduate deans, etc.) and/or the urgency of the staffing shortage (see DHSS, 1976). Table 6 shows the distribution by specialty of posts approved. Comparison with Table 4 shows that the

Table 6 Posts Approved in England and Wales under HM (69)6: 1 October 1971 to 15 April 1975

	Senior Registrar		Registrar	
Specialty	Number	% of total	Number	% of total
All Specialties	128	100	185	100
Medical Specialties	24	18.8	46	24.8
General Medicine	3	2.3	11	5.9
Paediatrics	8	6.3	13	7.0
Geriatrics	3	2.3	11	5.9
Surgical Specialties	0	0	0	0
Obstetrics and Gynaecology	0	0	3	1.0
Pathology	24	18.8	25	13.5
Anaesthetics	33	25.8	45	24.3
Radiology/Radiotherapy	14	10.9	12	6.5
Psychiatry	33	25.8	54	29.2

Source: DHSS Statistics and Research Division

posts are predominantly and hardly surprisingly, in 'women's fields', or to put it another way, in shortage specialties. (The number of posts in obstetrics and gynaecology is negligible, presumably because part-time training is not recognised.) This emphasis on particular specialities is encouraged officially.[17] Thus while these schemes have led to an increase in women's opportunities they have done so only on a limited scale and only in certain sectors of medicine. Restrictions on increases in medical staffing at all grades under the financial crisis of 1976 may paradoxically lead to an increase in the number of these special posts as they are unique in being 'sympathetically considered' officially (HM (69)6) by the appropriate authority.

Conclusion

This paper has suggested that analyses of the activity of women in medicine must go beyond explanations in terms of women's problems', i.e. the conflicting demands of home and work responsibilities. Such an approach cannot explain the variations in entry to medical school and in activity after qualification that have occurred.

Nor is an explanation in terms of role conflict reduction adequate to explain the concentration of women in particular sectors of medicine. Explanations in terms of discrimination in selection at medical school and in careers are insufficient, because these processes are themselves dependent on wider social practices. The concept of 'wastage', of under-utilisation of skilled womanpower is used as an argument for discrimination against women, but the assumptions underlying interpretation of women's wastage and working patterns are themselves problematic.

There has undoubtedly been a considerable increase in women doctors' opportunities in medicine, and this is likely to continue. However, this increase has taken place only in certain sectors of the highly structured medical labour market and women doctors have little influence over this structuring. Several recent developments have shown this. Because of the difficulties of attracting part-time staff into hospitals in clinical assistant posts with their unfavourable terms and conditions of service, a new grade of part-time hospital service post has been introduced, the hospital practitioner grade. This is restricted to principals in general practice so that a large number of holders of existing part-time posts, many of them women, are excluded from this new grade. Current legislative proposals include the introduction of mandatory three year vocational training for principals in general practice, for which no part-time provision (currently necessary, if unsatisfactory, for many women) was initially envisaged; only after protest is it now being considered.

In 1975 the provision of family planning was made a part of general practitioners' normal duties for which special payments were payable to the doctors. This has affected the opportunities for women doctors to be employed even in contraceptive clinics, the long-term prospects of which are now uncertain.

These changes are the outcome of negotiations between the government and the leaders of a profession, negotiations which have apparently failed to consider the position of women doctors. Rather than see women doctors as creating 'problems' for the medical staffing structure it may be more fruitful to look at the ways they are used to solve certain problems, problems not for the most part of their making.

Notes

1. This paper was prepared for a study of medical careers being carried out by Malcolm Johnson and myself funded by the SSRC. I should like to thank my colleagues in Leeds and at the Manchester Conference for their comments on the earlier version of this paper, and the DHSS Statistics and

Research Division for providing unpublished information.

2. As in other occupations women in medicine are concentrated in lower paid, lower status positions (see below and Epstein, 1970). The processes through which individual women are 'tracked out' of the prestigious specialties and posts, are not considered in detail in this paper. Lorber (1975) gives some suggestions as to possible processes but it is important to bear in mind that these processes themselves are rooted in the position of women in society as a whole. As Wolff has written, 'Organizational practices are very much integrated into and determined by social practice and ideological factors' (forthcoming, 1977).

3. 'Re-opening' is more appropriate because it is clear from historical and crosscultural studies that women have almost everywhere and at all times played the major part in all activities relating to the treatment of illness and the management of health. It is only in Western European and American Society since the nineteenth century that a single sex occupational group has dominated health care. (For historical accounts of the ousting of women practitioners from medicine, culminating in Britain in the 1858 Medical Act with its associated Register, see Ehrenreich and English, 1974; Donnison, 1977; Parry and Parry, 1976.) International studies show that in many countries women form a majority of doctors (e.g. Bowers, 1966) quite apart from forming the bulk of other employed health workers (Navarro, 1975b), and the vast army of mothers, wives, sisters and daughters who make up the hidden iceberg of unpaid health workers (Jefferys 1975).

4. For example, St Mary's, the last of the London schools to withdraw its facilities for women did so in 1924 because 'men for the most part preferred to go to a school where women were not taken' (Cope, 1963, p. 69). In 1929, following a University of London Senate statement that coeducation was desirable, the Dean of St Mary's said that they would take women *only* if all medical schools did so.

5. What evidence there is about women medical students' class origins suggest that they are recruited from a more exclusive social background than men. Navarro (1975a) has pointed out that the recent increase in the proportion of women (and blacks) in US medical schools has not been accompanied by an increase in the proportion of working-class students. The situation in Britain would appear to be similar.

6. Interviews with past and present deans and senior members of staff at medical schools confirm this. One former dean said that in his school during the late fifties and early sixties the entry criteria for men was 3 Cs (A level grades) but for women it was 2 Bs and a C: 'the standard had to be higher because of the pressure of applications.' At another school it was said that as early as 1959 the use of interviewing committees for selection was being queried, as, '. . . on interviews alone almost all students chosen should be girls. To some extent this was true for exam results as well . . . A 25% quota was operated . . . justified on the grounds that a female's life as a doctor was about 10 years compared to a man's 40.' Freidson suggests that the problem of women in the professions is of

> recruiting women who will stay in training and subsequently pursue a life-time career. Women are likely to be torn between a commitment to work and to marriage and family . . . Even in the case of that most professional of professions, medicine, only a modest proportion of women in the United States qualified to practise actually do so' (Freidson, 1970, p. 55).

The study quoted by Freidson (Dykeman and Stalnaker, 1957) shows of women graduating between 1925 and 1940 49 per cent were working full-time, and an additional 40 per cent were doing some medical work: not a very modest figure. The really modest proportion is surely that at the time of the study only 6 per cent of US medical students were women.

7. The recent increase in the number of applicants per place has raised the standard acceptable for both sexes, and the gap has narrowed. In October 1969 39 per cent of women students accepted at medical school had 3 B grades or higher, 23 per cent of men had similar grades. In 1973 50 per cent of women entrants had 3 Bs or higher, and 45 per cent of men. Applications from home candidates for medicine rose from 5.4 per cent of total applications in 1969 to 9.6 per cent in 1974. The proportion of admissions to medicine have not increased similarly. Medicine took 4.5 per cent of all admissions in 1969 and 4.9 per cent in 1974 (UCCA, 1975). *Source:* Table G *UCCA Statistical Supplements to Annual Reports.* Tables are based on a 10 per cent sample. Comparable data is only available for 1969 onwards.
8. The Willink Report erroneously held that women medical students' wastage rates were higher than men's. Jefferys *et al.* 1965 found that rates were identical though reasons for leaving different. Women show higher examination results at least in the pre-clinical years and are less likely to have to repeat years (Todd Report, 1968, Appendix 19).
9. Regarding women students the Todd Report noted the concern over the more stringent selection criteria applied to women but argued that 'the high proportion of women now accepted in some British medical schools is an indication that the admission of women to the course raises in itself few or no serious problems' (op. cit., para. 302, p. 123). The Todd Report refused to commit itself on whether or not women were likely to, or even should, make a greater contribution to medicine (see para. 356, p. 144) or whether any active steps should be taken to alter in any way the 'high' proportion (24 per cent) or the considerable variation between schools. In a full discussion of their position see Todd Report op. cit., p. 123.
10. The tone of this leader and many other articles on women doctors is reminiscent of the situation described by Rowbotham (1973):

    > Despite the dependence of capitalism now on married women as a permanent and essential part of the work force employers are still apt to behave as if they were going a favour by employing them. They still act as if women should somehow be grateful for the chance to be exploited. This is particularly ironic in view of the actual nature of the jobs which are categorised as 'women's work' (op. cit., p. 83).

    See the discussion on horizontal stratification of the medical labour market.
11. Analysis of professional working patterns tends to ignore questions of pay. It is often assumed that financial questions are not significant for women doctors because the principle of equal pay for men and women in the same posts is well established. Women doctors are concentrated in low paid posts but there is little information on the actual distribution of doctors' pay. Clinical assistant and other secondary sector posts are usually significantly disadvantaged in terms of fringe benefits relating to seniority payments, pensions, etc.
12. The progressive diminution in the proportion of women up the career hierarchy cannot be totally explained as a function of the recent increase in entry. The increase in the lower and non-training grades has been greater

than the increase in entry (as indicated by the almost constant proportion found in the pre-registration house posts). DHSS medical manpower figures exclude locum posts and as these are an important form of employment for women doctors, particularly in general practice, the figures underestimate the activity of women doctors.

13. These surveys analyse women's activities in terms of their life cycles. Because the surveys are non-comparable and are static, for the most part only referring to present activity, detailed reanalysis of data to show the kind of variations according to demand under the NHS suggested above is not possible. Looking at the changing patterns by ordering the various surveys chronologically supports the thesis of low activity during the fifties because of 'oversupply' and a steadily rising demand for 'pairs of hands' since the mid-sixties in all branches of medicine.
14. The provision of contraception is 'soul destroying' when the underutilisation of women doctors' skills is the question. When, however, proposals are made to allow such provision to be made by non-medically qualified personnel, e.g. insertion of IUDs and prescribing the 'pill' by nurses,it becomes a highly skilled task.
15. The Royal College of Psychiatrists and the Faculty of Anaesthetists were the first post-graduate educational bodies to recognise part-time training to relieve staff shortages. The Royal College of Surgeons and of Obstetricians and Gynaecologists have yet to do so.
16. These schemes are described in DHSS circulars, HM (69) 6 for part-time training in hospitals, ECN 564 for part-time employment in general practice, and HM (72) 74 for the Retainer Scheme. HM (69) 6 and HM (72) 74 are reproduced in DHSS 1976.
17. See the *BMJ* leader quoted above, 11 Jan. 1976, p. 56 and also p. 80 and DHSS 1976. Circulars have been issued by several Regional Health Authorities recommending that these posts only be created in shortage specialties.

References

Aird, L.A. and P.H.S. Silver (1971). ''Women doctors from the Middlesex Hospital Medical School (University of London) 1947-61', *BJME*, vol. 5, no. 3, pp. 232-41.

Barron, R.D. and G.M. Norris (1976). 'Sexual Divisions and the dual labour market', in D. Leonard Barker and S. Allen (eds.), *Sexual Divisions and Society: Process and Change.* London, Tavistock, pp. 47-49.

Beechey, V. 'Some Problems in the Analysis of Female Wage Labour in the Capitalist Mode of Production', paper given to *BSA* Sexual Division Study Group, May 1976.

Bell, C.S. (1975). 'The next revolution', *Social Policy,* Sept.-Oct. pp. 5-11.

Bell, E.M. (1953). *Storming the Citadel: The Rise of the Woman Doctor.* London, Constable.

Bewley, B.R. and T.H. Bewley, (1975). 'Hospital Doctors' Career Structure and Misuse of Medical Womanpower', *Lancet,* 9 August, pp. 270-73.

Blackstone, T. and O. Fulton. (1973). 'Sex differences, subject fields and research activity among academics in Britain and the United States', *9th Ann. Conf. of Society for Research into Higher Education,* Flood Page,C. & J. Gibson, (eds.)

pp. 36-68.
Blackstone, T. and O. Fulton (1975). 'Sex discrimination among University teachers: a British and American comparison', *Brit. J. Soc.*, vol. 26, no. 3, pp. 261-75.
Barker, D.L. and S. Allen. (1976a). Introduction to *Dependence and Exploitation in Work and Marriage,* London, Longmans, pp. 1-20.
Bowers, J. (1966). 'Women in medicine, an international study', *New Eng. J. Med.*, vol. 275, pp. 362-5.
Bowlby, J. (1952). 'Maternal Care and Mental Health', *World Health Organisation Bulletin No. 3,* Geneva, WHO.
British Medical Association (1948). *The Training of a Doctor.* London BMA.
Community Relations Commission (1976). *Doctors from Overseas, A Case for Consultation.* London.
Cope, Z. (1963). *The History of St. Mary's Medical School.* London, Heinemann.
Davies, R. (1975). *Woman and Work,* London, Arrow.
Department of Health and Social Security (1969). Circular HM (69)6, Employment of Women Doctors in Hospital Service.
Department of Health and Social Security (1976). *Women in Medicine,* Proceedings of Conference organised by DHSS, 4-5 July 1975, Sunningdale.
Donnison, J. (1977). *Midwives and Medical Men.* London, Heinemann Educational.
Dykman, R.A. and J.M. Stalnaker. (1957). 'Survey of women physicians graduating from medical school 1925-1940', *J.M. Educ.*, vol. 32, no. 3, pp. 3-38.
Eckstein, H. (1960). *Pressure Group Politics.* London, George Allen & Unwin.
Ehrenreich, B. and D. English (1974). *Witches, Midwives and Nurses; A History of Women Healers.* Old Westbury, New York, Feminist Press.
Elston, M.A. (1977). 'Medical Autonomy: the Challenge and Response', in K.A.B. Barnard and K. Lee (eds.), *Conflict in the National Health Service.* London, Croom Helm.
Epstein, C.F. (1970). *Woman's place: options and limits in professional careers,* Berkeley, Calif., Univ. of Calif. Press.
Flynn, C.A. and F. Gardner. (1969). 'The careers of women graduates from the Royal Free Hospital School of Medicine, London', *BJME,* vol. 3, no. 1, pp. 28-42.
Fogarty, M.P.,R. and R.N. Rapoport. (1972). *Sex, Career and Family.* London, George Allen-Unwin for PEP.
Freidson, E. (1970). *Profession of Medicine.* New York, Dodd, Mead & Co.
Goodenough Report (1944). *Report of the Inter-Departmental Committee on Medical Schools.* London, HMSO.
Holter, H. (1971). 'Sex roles and social change', *Acta. Sociol.*, vol. 14, pp. 2-12.
Jefferys, M. (1966). 'Marriage, motherhood and medicine', *Transactions of the Sixth World Congress of Sociology,* vol. IV, Sept. 1966. ISA.
Jefferys, M. (1975). 'Women in health: A view from Europe', *Int. Conf. on Women in Health,* 16 June, Pan American Health Organisation, Washington, D.C.
Jefferys, M. S. Gauvain and O. Gulesen. (1965). 'Comparison of men and women in medical training', *Lancet,* vol. 1. pp. 1381-3.
Jefferys, M. and P.M. Elliot (1966). *Women in Medicine.* London, Office of Health Economics.
Johnson, T.J. (1972). *Professions and Power.* London, Macmillan Press.
Kelsall, R.K.,A. Poole and A. Kuhn (1972). *Graduates: The Sociology of an Elite.* London, Methuen.
Kosa, J. and R.E. Coker (1965). 'The female physician in public health, conflict and reconciliation of the sex and professional roles', *Sociology and Social*

Research, vol. 49, no. 3, pp. 296-7.
Lorber J. (1975). 'Women and Medical Sociology: Invisible Professionals and Ubiquitous Patients', in M. Millman and R.M. Kanter (eds.), *Another Voice: Feminist Perspectives on Social Life and Social Science.* New York, Anchor, pp. 73-105.
Lopate, C. 1968). *Women in Medicine.* Baltimore, Johns Hopkins University Press.
Merrison Report (1957). *Report of the Committee of Inquiry into the regulation of the medical professions.* London, HMSO, Cmnd. 6018.
Navarro, V. (1975a). 'The Political Economy of Health Care', *Int. Jnl. Health Services,* vol. 5, no. 1. pp. 65-94.
Navarro, V. (1975b). 'Women in health care', *New England Journal of Medicine,* vol. 292, no. 8, pp. 398-402.
Oakley, A. (1974). *Housewife.* London, Allen Lane.
Ogston, D., A.A. Dawson and G.M. McAndrew. (1969). 'Present employment of University of Aberdeen medical graduates 1965-68', *Lancet,* vol. 2, pp. 427-8.
Parry N. and J. Parry. (1976). *The Rise of the Medical Profession.* London, Croom Helm.
Parkin, F. (1974). 'Strategies of Social Change in Class Formation', in F. Parkin, (ed.), *The Social Analysis of Class Structure.* London, Tavistock, pp. 1-18.
Parsons, T. (1951). *The Social System.* London, Routledge & Kegan Paul, ch. 10.
Rossi, A.S. (1964). 'Equality between the sexes: an immodest proposal', *Daedalus,* vol. 93, Spring, pp. 607-52.
Rowbotham, S. (1973). *Woman's Consciousness: Man's World.* London, Penguin.
Shaw, J. (1976). 'Finishing School: Some Implications of Sex-Segregated Education' in D.L. Barker and S. Allen, (1976b) (eds.), *Sexual Divisions and Society: Process and Change,* London, Tavistock, pp. 133-49.
Smith R. (1976). 'Sex and Occupational role on Fleet Street', in Barker and Allen, 1976a, op. cit., pp. 70-87.
Todd Report (1968). *Report of Royal Commission on Medical Education.* London, HMSO, Cmnd. 3569.
Ulyatt, K.W. and F.M. Ulyatt. (1970). 'Field and training performance of a group of women doctors', *The Medical Officer,* vol. 124, pp. 33-4.
Whitfield, A.G.N. (1969). 'Women Medical Graduates of the University of Birmingham 1959-63', *BMJ,* 5 July, pp. 44-6.
Willink Report, 1957, *Report of the Committee on Inquiry to consider the future number of medical practitioners and the appropriate intake of students.* London, HMSO.
Wolff, J. (1977). 'Women in Organisations', in S. Clegg and D. Dunkerley (ed.), *Critical Issues in Organisation.* London, Routledge & Kegan Paul.

Like several of the papers in this volume, Nigel Goldie's analysis of the division of labour among the medical and paramedical workers in mental health concentrates closely on the everyday work situation of rank and file members of the occupations involved. The pronouncements of occupational leaders, spokesmen and ideologists are seen to offer data only on their own problems and their own situations. Their link with everyday practice is an empirical question.

Goldie's central problem is that of reconciling the 'objective' powerlessness and lack of autonomy of psychologists and social workers with their 'subjective' unawareness of their own impotence in relation to psychiatrists. He shows that it is not possible to treat each occupation as homogenous and that this segmentation generates certain types of accommodation to the problem of securing professional status without either power or autonomy. In each occupation some groups define their situation as one of ancillary workers to the psychiatrists, where they have a distinct but subordinate part to play under medical leadership. Others define their situation as one of complementing the psychiatrists, where the boundaries of appropriate occupational work are blurred and doctors are assigned a coordinating rather than a directive role; finally, others adopt an anti-psychiatry position, opposing the whole notion of any hierarchical division of labour.

Nevertheless, particular institutions can absorb a good deal of variation, partly because psychiatrists are themselves divided along similar lines and partly because of a reality constraint. The paramedical workers can sustain their own position by a process of self-limitation, regarding themselves as 'free' within 'realistic' limits set by the psychiatrists' legal and other responsibilities. The psychiatrists themselves consequently find few grounds for forcing the issue, besides being subject to everyday interactional constraints of tact and politeness.

This paper offers an interesting attempt to move micro sociological work into an analysis of structural issues. It may well be, in the long run, that this is a more profitable line of development than seeking an uneasy coexistence or synthesis between constructivist and interpretive approaches. One of the major challenges facing our discipline as a whole is that of providing empirically grounded statements on traditional issues, like class, status and power, in terms which can articulate with observable social action and the interpretive frames with which actors order that action. Goldie's approach is an early example of a burgeoning field of enquiry.

R.D. and M.E.R.

THE DIVISION OF LABOUR AMONG THE MENTAL HEALTH PROFESSIONS – A NEGOTIATED OR AN IMPOSED ORDER?

Nigel Goldie

The aim of this paper is to raise certain questions about the study of interprofessional relationships in work locales shared by 'rival' professions. The perspective used in the study will first be examined and certain points made about the occupations of psychiatry, clinical psychology and social work. The ideologies discerned among the members of these occupations are then considered. This provides a context in which to place the substantive material of the paper, namely the nature of the autonomy enjoyed by social workers and clinical psychologists. Finally, the analysis raises various questions about the nature of the social structure of interprofessional relations, and the role of ideology in the study of these relations.

Introduction

The literature on professions and professionalisation is extensive.[1] There is a large number of empirical studies of professionalisation of various occupations and discussions of the theoretical questions which this process raises.[2] This literature has been critically reviewed several times in recent years, and rather than reiterating the now widely accepted criticisms of the 'trait' and 'functionalist' views of professionalisation, it is more important to note the assumptions that have informed this paper's approach. First, it is believed that professions can be differentiated from other occupations by their generally higher salaries, status and legal privileges. The possession of (or seeking after) these and other attributes should not obscure the more fundamental question of how the members of a profession attempt to gain and preserve control over the practice of certain activities.[3] In this respect professions are no different from other occupations that seek autonomy over their own affairs. Professions, however, are generally those occupations that have been successful at preventing the encroachment of rival groups who claim expertise to practise in the same areas as themselves. Thus 'professionalisation' is rarely, if ever, seen to occur in a social vacuum, but is accomplished and sustained in the face of these rival claims. There is, therefore, a need to situate this process within the institutions in which the various rivals work out a division of labour between themselves. Further, it is believed that the meaning of professionalisation may be quite different to the membership of a profession compared with the aims, ambitions and activities of the various officeholders and 'spokesmen' of a particular professional association. Finally it is necessary to study the ideological differences found within and between different professional groups. These ideologies reflect the interests of the group concerned to maintain control over both the practice of their particular expertise and various aspects of their 'work space'. Views on the legitimacy of the hierarcy within and between the various occupations are important elements in such ideologies. Within the context of the mental health professions, such ideologies are likely to centre around differing views on the aetiology and treatment of mental illness.[4] However, while it is necessary to be aware of the differences in outlook towards treatment, the more important differences may be seen in the way staff understand and view the social structure of the treatment setting in which they work.

A summary of the main ideological types discerned during a study of psychiatrists, social workers and clinical psychologists will be made before going on to consider the main focus of the paper, the way in which the division of labour is negotiated within the social structure of their institutions. One of the main problems encountered is that of the evident differences in the insitutional power of the occupations concerned, while the members of these occupations deny that such differpences in any way limit their freedom and autonomy. This paper is therefore concerned with the complex task of reconciling certain 'objective' features of the social structure of treatment settings found within mental hospitals, with the 'subjective' views of these features as held by the staff who were interviewed. It is argued here that although there is a danger of entering an 'infinite regress' and of retreating into subjectivism, attention has to be paid to the way that actors themselves define their own situation, and how their actions, intentions and motivations form a dialectic with the institutions in which they participate. However, institutions such as mental hospitals have long histories, and their pasts continue to influence their present in many ways. There are also various contingencies and 'institutional imperatives', from within and without the hospital, that have a considerable influence on the organisation structure to be found within any particular hospital.[5] The nature of the catchment area, the resources and facilities available within the hospital and its catchment area, the demand for beds and the legal requirements upon the 'responsible medical officer', can all be seen to exert an influence over the activities of staff within any particular hospital. While to some degree negotiable, such features clearly provide an 'objective' structure for the institutions in which the mental health occupations are located.

These occupations – psychiatry, clinical psychology and social work – have received a certain amount of attention from sociologists in the United States, but very little in this country.[6] In consequence, we face the problem of drawing from ideas, findings and theories developed in another cultural context. The American literature on these professions, for example, presents a picture of considerable conflict and professional rivalry, both between individual practitioners in their workplaces and between the various professional associations.[8] The members of the lay professions are generally presented as seeking greater professional recognition and taking a combative approach towards the psychiatrists, while the latter, in turn, seek to restrict the former, and prevent encroachment.[8] While such conflict may, in part, have an economic base (being over private practice patients), it may also owe its origins to the administrative structure within American hospitals.[9] It is also the case that all three occupations appear to be claiming unique skills in psychotherapy as their main therapeutic contribution.[10] I have argued elsewhere that in the British context, the nature of the medical mandate being claimed by psychiatrists is more concerned with incorporating lay staff than excluding them.[11] I have also pointed out that the 'liberalism' shown by psychiatrists towards lay staff, enables the latter to accommodate themselves to the *status quo*[12]. In the context of the earlier discussion on professionalisation, it should be noted that both social work and clinical psychology can be seen to be 'professionalising' occupations, in so far as they are adopting the various attributes of a profession, such as a register of members, codes of ethics, standardised training and so forth. However, it is apparent that within both occupations there are serious divisions of opinion over the nature of the skills possessed by their members.[13] Further, while social workers have gained greater control over their own affairs in local authorities, following the Seebohm reorganisation, they, along with psychologists and other lay staff, have remained subordinate to the medical profession in mental hospitals.

While it is not the concern of this paper to pass judgement on whether or not social work, clinical psychology or psychiatry are 'professions', it is worth noting the comment of Freidson (1971) that, 'a dominant profession stands in an entirely different structural relationship to the division of labour than does a subordinate profession'

(p. 137). Freidson (1970) has also argued that it is having *autonomy* over one's actions, as he claims the medical profession has, that defines a 'genuine' profession. Freidson's case is a strong one, even if one may object to the attempt to find a single criterion with which to distinguish professions from other occupations. However, certain criticisms can be levelled at this view of the medical profession being 'all powerful'. At one level there is the view that the state is increasingly regulating the affairs of the medical profession,[14] while at a more micro level, there is the view that doctors have to 'work' continually at maintaining their autonomy. From ethnomethodology, several studies have shown how doctors adopt various 'routines' and 'strategies' in the daily ordering of various 'emergencies' in order to preserve their autonomy in the face of various challenges from patients, relatives and other staff.[15]

From a different theoretical perspective, symbolic interactionism, other points of criticism have emerged. In a series of papers, a group of American sociologists have published accounts of the work of various professions in medical and related contexts.[16] In a paper that draws together the implications of much of this earlier work, Bucher and Stelling (1969), have argued that the social structure of the work situation of professionals in organisations such as mental hospitals is one in which there is continuous negotiation and renegotiation. They argue that in such work locales there is no pre-existing role structure, 'Rather the new member builds his own place in the organisation and creates the role he plays there' (p. 5). Further, 'Role creation is a direct consequence of being accorded professional status. The professional is the person who has the right to say what should be done and what is necessary to get it done' (p. 5). Other points flow from these assertions; 'professionals' seek to control their 'work space', and their 'self-esteem, reputation, and career' are at stake. Having outlined the various forms that 'negotiation' takes at an individual level, Bucher and Stelling consider it at the collective level. They note how there is 'continually unfolding internal differentiation or segmentalisation within the organisation' (p. 7). They liken this process to a political one, involving negotiation, bargaining and the formation and dissolution of alliances. The consequence being that 'the power to determine policy is not clearly located in specific positions. It is more diffuse, and the locus and balance of power often shifts in response to different issues, and as different groups and persons move through the organisation' (p. 11). Not only is 'power' seen to be 'diffuse', but it becomes largely a matter of 'interpersonal influence'. While this perspective is open to certain criticisms for its neglect of the prior domination and power of certain groups,[17] Bucher and Stelling have made an important contribution by drawing attention to the complexity of this issue, and the danger of simply reducing the question of authority relations between professions to a zero-sum formulation.

Thus there is a need, on the one hand, to consider the question of autonomy as a key to any discussion of professionalisation, while, on the other, there is the need to consider the possibility that mental hospitals are 'arenas' in which there are shifting balances of power. The question then becomes one of how to account for the objective differences in power that can be observed to structure relationships with the subjective awareness and denials of such differences. I shall attempt to deal with this by examining the different ideologies that were found in interviews with clinical and non-clinical staff and, the nature of the autonomy enjoyed by or denied to the lay staff. Unlike Bucher and Stelling, who appear to claim that power cannot be identified and located, it is believed that the medical profession is still in a structurally dominant position in British mental hospitals. Further, in contrast to Freidson who appears to assert that staff either have complete autonomy or none at all, it is believed that it is very difficult to identify the nature of 'autonomy', without reference to the way that staff themselves perceived the extent of their own freedom.

The Ideologies

The material to be presented in this paper is drawn from interviews with thirty-eight psychiatrists, thirty-eight social workers and twenty-seven clinical psychologists.[18] The interview guide consisted of open-ended questions mainly about the respondents' views of their work, their relationships with other staff, their awareness of direction and their views on mental illness and its treatment.[19] Clearly there are many problems to be overcome when carrying out the type of research from which this data is drawn, not the least being that of seeking the confidence of 'rival' groups and of moving between them in such a way that the researcher is not identified with any particular group.[20] Quite apart from such difficulties there is the question of the way a person will represent their views on matters that may affect their professional and personal self-conceptions to an outsider. Clearly all interviews, whatever their purpose, are highly problematic affairs, involving the social construction of a negotiated outcome, namely the eventual written record of what was said.

It was during the stage when interviews were being analysed that the ideologies to be described 'emerged'. That is, various interconnections were discerned between what was said in reply to certain questions and it became apparent that replies to certain questions could only be understood when considered as a part of the totality of a particular person's world view or ideology. The schema of the points of contrast between the ideologies shown in Figure 1, provides some indication of the wide range of these interconnections. The subsequent quotations

Figure 1 Schema of Points of Contrast between the Ideologies*

Area of contrast	Welfare Worker Doctor Tester	Therapist Eclectics Professional	Dissident
Expertise/tasks	Exclusive/limited	Inclusive/broad ranging	Limited/ denigrating
Division of labour	Clear cut/overlap at edges	Blurring/overlap at centre	Should be complete over-lap
View of other staff's role	Restrictive	Liberal	Liberal
View of psychi-atrists (by lay staff)	Superior knowledge/ leadership/treatment	Limited knowledge/ coordination/treat psychoses only	Rejection of medical model but accept drugs
Mental illness as medical problem	Almost entirely	Equivocal	No
Treatment	Drugs/physical & practical care	Use drugs, but psychotherapy as *real* therapy	Live through experience and learn from it
Psychiatrist's authority	Legitimate	Mixed	Illegitimate
Awareness of direction	Little, if any	Some – not restrictive	Aware and resentful
Disagreement with other staff	Rarely, if ever	Sometimes	Frequently
Own relevance	Yes, important	Yes, could/should be more so	Very little
Attitudes to own profession (by lay staff)	Mixed – anti-professionalisation	Pro- keen to professionalise	Anti- critical of own profession
Attitudes to training	Practical experience	Academic	Personal knowledge
Relations with patients	Distance/ neutrality	Mixed – be person and transference figure	Involvement with patient
Collective action	Mixed	Mixed	Keen – if ineffective

*The left-hand column of areas of contrast provides some indication of some of the issues that were specifically raised during the interviews. Such schemas always tend to oversimplify; its purpose is to illustrate how the ideologies contain many varied elements.

serve to illustrate the points of contrast. As the focus of this paper is not the ideologies themselves, the picture that is presented of them must inevitably be a superficial one.[21] For the purposes of this paper the 'welfare worker' ideology identified among the social workers has been grouped together with that of the 'doctors' and 'testers' found among the psychiatrists and clinical psychologists respectively. Similarly the 'therapist' ideology from among the social workers is considered along with the 'eclectic' and 'professional' ideologies from the other occupations. Finally, the dissident ideology is considered to be common to all three occupations and thus is treated as such. The main points of contrast between the three types of ideology can be seen in the schema of elements. I have analysed all of the ideologies in detail elsewhere, and all that will be given here are a few quotations to illustrate particular facets of them.[22]

Thus taking the first category of ideologies, there were 'doctors' who would assert that:

> I see my task to be dealing with the primarily medical aspects of things. As a psychiatrist one is first and foremost a doctor and so is dealing with the medical aspects of the situation. I disagree with those colleagues who think they have a divine right to take part in all aspects of the patients' care. There are other staff who are more capable than us at some things and we should let them get on with it (1506).[23]

The welfare worker ideology, while stressing the importance of the value of the practical assistance to be given patients, contains a similar view on the need to avoid overlap or 'role blurring', as well as recognition of the more important role of the psychiatrist whose tasks were seen to be: 'Diagnosis, treatment, deciding upon admissions, using all the various ancillaries. In the treatment of psychiatric illness he is the king-pin. His essential role is to diagnose and delegate treatment in the appropriate way' (3206). Thus while seeing themselves as playing an 'auxiliary role', there is also a view of mental illness as 'an illness that ought to be curable, and it ought to be preventable as other illnesses are'. Such views were reflected in comments from the testers as to the indispensibility of medical treatments. As one of them put it, 'Just imagine what this hospital would be like without the doctors to prescribe the drugs. Wards that were like bedlam twenty years ago are now as hushed as cathedrals' (2600). Within this first category of ideologies, there is a general affirmation of the need for medical direction and an assumption that this is both natural and appropriate. One welfare worker illustrates: 'I know my limitations, I don't agree at all with those social workers who think they are the GPs of psychiatry and can take over as therapists' (3211). By way of contrast the second category of ideologies contained claims such as those of one 'professional' psychologist that:

> A psychologist is an independent specialist while his role is a matter of negotiation. Not conscious negotiation, but the give and take of interpersonal relationships. I think that the psychologist who ignores that the doctor is in charge is making a grave mistake which might even be harmful. It's not a clear cut answer, but its not a clear cut situation (2900).

Other psychologists listed a wide range of activities that they could be involved in while stressing how their expertise embraced 'much more than testing'. This tendency to dissassociate oneself from the more traditional activities was also paralleled among the therapist social workers and the eclectic psychiatrists. Thus in so far as members of all three occupations claimed to be able to give 'therapy', 'psychotherapy' and to be able to offer 'insights' to patients, it was recognised that there was an overlap. As one eclectic psychiatrist put it:

> The roles are not clearly defined, this in itself does not matter, as an interdisciplinary approach is where the borders on one's knowledge and training merge with that of the others. So while the others expect the doctor to be more knowledgeable about the psychiatric states and the psychodynamic conflicts that the patient has everyone has insights into the patient and the community. In the end though because of the responsibility of the doctor, and the doctor has the final responsibility for the care of patients, the other staff expect him to make a more important contribution (151).

This quotation illustrates the apparent 'liberalism' of the eclectic ideology, an ideology that contains various assertions about the supremacy of medical knowledge and the need for medical 'leadership' if not 'direction'. In their perspective the lay staff recognise the need to be 'realistic' and accept the legal responsibility of the psychiatrists, while harbouring desires for a less medically-dominated system and denying the psychiatrists' claims. As one psychologist observed: 'Well apart from pushing drugs into people, which is necessary, and only they can do, most of the rest could be done by other members of the staff, just as well, if not better. At least social workers and psychologists are not hidebound by a narrow medical education' (2505). The ideologies of both the 'professional' and the 'therapist' stress how it is possible to achieve good working relations with certain psychiatrists, if the correct approach is taken. Such a process of accommodation enables them to pursue their therapeutic ambitions with neurotic or drug addicted patients, while leaving 'the schizophrenics, the psychotics, endogenous depressions and the hysterical patients as medical problems, but not the neurotics or personality disorders' (3507). As might be expected, among the lay staff the ideologies of the 'professional' and the 'therapists' stress the need to professionalise their occupations. Thus the respective professional associations are expected to be 'protecting' and advancing the interests of their members in various ways as well as establishing registers and the other attributes of professional status.

By way of contrast with the other ideological types, the dissidents, as the term implies,expressed various discordant views of both own occupation and colleagues and the current structure of the mental health services. In order to illustrate the general tenor of the claims being made by the dissidents the following quotations are provided:

> You don't need to be medically qualified or to have a knowledge of academic psychology to understand what happens when a person breaks down. It's much more a matter of who you are rather than what you are. The real work in a place like this is being your real self with patients. If you can't stand suffering then you are no good – you cannot help anybody (2802).

Alongside a critique of professionalism in general, there were other claims that go against conventional practices. For example one dissident psychiatrist said:

> I might consider sleeping with a patient, but this would depend on what seems appropriate. If it helps toward understanding the person as a person, in their own terms, instead of in some psychiatric category, then it means getting involved with them. I can learn from them as well as they from me (1511).

Other elements of the dissident ideology involved a 'restrictive' view of their own expertise as well as that of the other staff, and frequent assertions as to their current 'irrelevant', 'messenger boy' or 'technician' role. The dissidents were much more aware of being directed or controlled by the medical profession. As one social worker observed: 'The doctors are a sort of blockage, they prevent me doing the sort of things that I would like to be doing' (3503). There were also assertions about the role that they, along with the other staff, played in social control. The influence of the anti-psychiatrists, especially the work of R.D. Laing, was evident in their views on 'mental illness' and the most appropriate forms of therapy. As one psychologist commented:

> Being 'mad' should be a way of life that can be considered feasible for those that want it. I find it very disturbing how doctors and 'eminent' people can act as experts in deciding how people should live . . . what we need are small units or sanctuaries or retreats, where people know there is some sort of knowledge and experience for them (2503).

While other staff who were critical of their working situations appeared to be able to find justifications for continuing to work in the mental health services, the dissidents were more likely to express a sense of futility and to indicate that they would be likely to cease working before long.

The ideological types have been introduced in order to illustrate the differences in outlook and motivation on the part of the membership of these three occupations. They also serve a wider purpose in introducing several issues that should be noted before considering the actual question of the nature of the autonomy enjoyed by the social workers and clinical psychologists. In particular, it is clear that the nature of the 'professional challenge' posed by the social workers and the clinical psychologists is not one of united occupations seeking to extend their mandates, but rather of loose groups of individuals who have differing conceptions as to the expertise they possess and the role they should play. Similarly the expectations that psychiatrists hold of lay staff differ, even if there is overall acceptance of the necessity for 'team work' and the involvement of lay staff in the treatment process. The analysis of the ideologies also shows differences in the way that the division of labour is viewed. When asked specifically about this, the psychiatrists as a whole were much more likely to consider it to be both 'natural' and 'clear cut', whereas both the social workers and clinical psychologists were more likely to claim there were large areas of overlap between the work of the several occupations. Obviously this assertion should be qualified by reference to the ideological types, for the therapists and professionals were more likely than the testers and welfare workers to claim to be able to practice psychotherapy, as well, as, if not better than, the psychiatrists. It would require a separate paper to explore all the issues relating to the nature of psychotherapy and the qualifications required to practice it; all that can be said here is that most of those interviewed claimed that ability as a 'therapist' depended on qualities of personality more than anything else. The implications of this for the future professionalisation of both social work and clinical psychology will be noted later.

Before doing this, however, it is necessary to introduce further material on the structural position of the lay staff. This will be approached through consideration of the nature of the referral process and the degree to which social workers and psychologists had problems in gaining access to the patients that interested them. The ability of psychiatrists to prevent lay staff from having access to certain patients is regarded as an example of their 'objective' power. The extent to which this power is actually seen as restrictive and limiting, though, will depend on the sort of contact the lay staff wish to have with patients which may be quite limited, as we have said above.

Referrals to the Social Workers and Psychologists and their Problems of Gaining Access to Patients

In Rushings' (1964) study the social workers and, to a lesser extent, the psychologists, found gaining access to patients to be one of their major problems. Clearly the basis on which staff gain access to patients not only largely defines what they are able to do with patients, but also determines the extent to which their performance is judged by other staff. Freidson (1971) has drawn attention to the way that specialists, who are dependent on colleagues for referrals, must be mindful of the criteria of performance of those colleagues, if they are to ensure a steady supply of patients. Referral processes can be considered to provide at least an outline of the structure of relationships between the medical and lay occupations.

Perhaps as a reflection of the greater acceptance of the social workers by the psychiatrists, only a few social workers reported any problems in gaining access to patients. With the possible exception of the two working at Oakdene Hospital, all the other hospital social workers noted how their involvement as 'members of a team' gave them direct access to any of the patients on their units. The situation of the psychologists was less clear cut, as they were only attached to certain teams at Wheatbury and Willows Hospital. Even in these hospitals the psychologists also received referrals in the traditional manner, while the remainder were in the position of one psychologist who commented: 'We do not get access to patients to see them for ourselves, but only when they are sent to us by the doctor. I am not in a position to pick out patients for therapy, except as a by-product of a referral' (2505). Other psychologists however, stressed how they had a 'free hand' in being able to see whatever patients interested them. The significance of this question of access, when considering the nature of the autonomy enjoyed by the lay staff, becomes apparent in a comment from one of the principal psychologists: 'The doctors can stop us doing things, they control who comes here, we cannot demand to see patients – but that's about all – they can limit us in that way' (2500). In this and other ways, psychologists would frequently introduce the fact of the psychiatrists' ultimate control over their access to patients. It was noted earlier that the various welfare tasks carried out by most social workers have made them essential for the smooth running of admission units in mental hospitals. This may account for the readier access that they had to patients than that enjoyed by the psychologists. Certainly many psychologists drew attention to their dependence on certain psychiatrists for 'interesting referrals', and in some cases for patients at all. The dependent position of such psychologists can be well illustrated by reference to one particular psychologist, who considered himself a qualified psychotherapist but had no direct access to patients. He pointed out:

> I was receiving patients on a regular basis from a consultant who has just left. He trusted me and his leaving has been a great set back to me. I was taking both individual and group psychotherapy with his patients, but this has all stopped. This stems from the instability of the whole organisation. One day I feel that things are going very well and that I have a central role, but then the next day I find that the consultant or registrar have left, and so I have to start all over again (2601).

This psychologist was, admittedly, in a difficult position as the only one in a 1,600 bed hospital, but he was not alone in finding himself in a situation where he had to depend on the favours of individual psychiatrists, to gain access to patients that he felt he could help. Many of those psychologists who worked in situations where they had more direct access also felt their contribution was affected, if not wholly determined, by the nature of the relationship that they enjoyed with certain psychiatrists within the teams of which they were members. Throughout the interviews there were frequent references to this problem. It should be noted that psychologists upholding all three types of ideologies drew attention to it in various ways. Such psychologists clearly felt that what they could do with patients depended very much on who the referring agent was. In contrast, very few social workers drew attention to this problem, although several mentioned how some psychiatrists were more directive and specific than others when requesting that they do something.

The situation of the social workers was in some ways more complicated than that of the psychologists. They were expected to attend ward rounds, staff meetings and other occasions when decisions affecting patients were made. Although they were present at such decisions and thus potentially able to affect them in a way that was often denied to the psychologists, the extent to which they still had to wait for patients to be referred *to* them, remains far from clear. For example many of the 'welfare workers' conveyed the impression of knowing what was required of them and thus they would not wait for a specific referral. Other social workers noted how they were 'requested to do things', or as one of them said:

> There is quite a lot of medical direction, since most of the things that I do are referred from ward rounds. But what I do after that is up to me. A doctor may suggest that I see a patient's husband, but they don't tell me what to say. It's hard to tell whether its direction or co-operation – it doesn't feel like direction to me (3601).

One of the 'therapists' observed how 'some of the social workers let themselves become the handmaiden of the doctors' and then pointed out: 'I initiate referrals myself, this is where my approach is different, I suggest where social work is necessary, whereas many wait until it is asked for' (3511). However, another social worker on the same unit noted that, 'I am asked to do things, and they are expected to be done, but how and when is up to me' (3512). Many social workers claimed that they were able to ignore, reinterpret or modify requests made to them by the doctors, or as one of them observed, 'it is very easy to manipulate the situation here' (3507). This was especially the case where the social workers only saw the consultants infrequently. The significance of these remarks is not the varied ways of coping with referrals, but, rather, the choice of tactical means of resistance, avoiding a direct confrontation with the psychiatrists. Although some of the staff did make reference to certain problems in gaining access to particular types of patients, none saw the problem to be an insurmountable one.[24] In contrast to the social workers of Rushings' (1964) study who had the problems of routinising referrals to themselves, in this study it was another group, the psychologists, who had the greater problems. But there were many references to having to discourage certain kinds of referrals that were considered unnecessary or demeaning.[25]

The question of autonomy, however, cannot be left with the issue of gaining access to patients, for, as some of the quotations suggested, there were members of both occupations who felt themselves to be 'directed' from time to time by the psychiatrists. This 'freedom' can lead to a certain amount of mystification and encourage the belief that one has autonomy over one's own actions. This is especially the case in a therapeutic community and when members of staff have limited and circumscribed conceptions of their own tasks and role. Bearing in mind the way that many psychiatrists seek to be non-directive in their relations with ancillary staff, it is hardly surprising that there should be frequent observations, such as one made by a social worker that, 'There is direction, but not supervision over how you actually do the work' (3604)

The Lay Staff's Awareness of Direction and Supervision

As the final short quotation above demonstrates, many of the social workers drew a distinction between being directed as opposed to being supervised. This distinction did not appear to be anywhere near so important for the psychologists, who rarely referred to there being direction over how they worked. What was more important for the psychologists was the nature of the relationship they had with *particular* psychiatrists, and the extent to which this 'limited' or 'restricted' their contribution. But at the same time nearly all the lay staff offered conflicting definitions of their professional limits. An important element in the 'professional' ideology was the representation of their relationships with the psychiatrists in terms that suggested they were not limited in what they did. A central assumption within this ideology is the emphasis on 'working within realistic limits', in order to maintain autonomy over what one does within such limits. At the same time, however, psychologists were usually very much aware of the fact that the psychiatrists had more power than themselves. They tended to accept this as inevitable, and only complained of excessive or arbitrary use of this power. Such awareness was shown by one psychologist who said:

> The fact of the doctors having legal responsibility does affect the kind of things that you can carry out. But I am happy to carry out those kinds of things, as I find them useful for the patients and moderately interesting. I quite like the work that I am doing so I think this is alright. I am very happy for them to have the legal responsibility (2902).

What is signficant about this quotation is the way the fact of legal responsibility is introduced, for, as another psychologist commented, 'You are continually being made aware that you are dealing with someone else's responsibility' (2095). Clearly, this legal responsibility cannot be 'negotiated' beyond a certain point, and it remains as a continual reminder to the lay staff of their inferior position. As was pointed out in the earlier analysis of the ideologies, there are some lay staff, especially the 'welfare workers' and the 'testers', who believed that it was right that the psychiatrists should have this responsibility, but others saw no reason why they should not also share these responsibilities. Thus, on the one hand, there was an overall affirmation by the majority of lay staff that they had considerable freedom. This was especially the case among the staff working in therapeutic community contexts with their accent on 'communication' and 'participation', such that everyone is asked their opinion, while no one is told what to do. On the other hand, there was an awareness of being 'limited' or 'directed' or of 'feeling accountable' that many felt in various direct and indirect ways. Frequently this awareness amounted to a form of self-limitation that could arise from 'being aware of a certain ethos, and not stepping outside it' (2904), or from such experiences as those recounted by a psychologist at Oakdene:

> I am aware of some constraints, we have to make sure that the doctors agrees before taking a particular course of treatment with a patient. Otherwise we are given a free hand. But being aware of particular difficulties, I don't take certain people on for therapy. Some of the treatment that we have given in the past has been sabotaged by the doctors and nurses, so we now really only do counselling work. We have a lot to offer, but we know it won't work in the present set up, so we don't bother trying (2042).

However, more typical were comments like that of a 'therapist' social worker, 'I am very free, although I do have to justify what I do to the doctors. This comes under the pretence of so-called feedback, but is not overpowering or restrictive' (3509). Sometimes such self-limitation took the form of not engaging in certain activities for fear of being rebuffed, or as one social worker observed; 'I am very cautious about taking patients on for psychotherapy, although I have had experience of carrying it out in my previous local authority job. I am almost fearing the doctors' disapproval, though for myself I don't think the limits are very tight' (3506).

This process of self-limitation is similar to other tendencies noted among the lay staff that took the form of holding a 'restricted' or 'narrow' view of one's own expertise and tasks. Through such a process a 'working consensus' is arrived at, over who should do what, without any apparent bargaining or negotiation taking place. It is merely assumed by all parties concerned that certain staff carry out certain activities. Clearly disputes do arise, but what seems to be more remarkable is the reported accord or agreement that appears to exist. Apart from those lay staff who were actually aware of such 'limitations', others who drew attention to 'hidden' pressures. As one social worker commented, 'It's all hidden pressure, it's only when you don't do something over a long period that you find the pressure.' Significantly, it was the dissidents who most frequently drew attention to such pressure, for it was they who most frequently transgressed the assumptions about the limits of their appropriate contribution. One such social worker for example reported having:

> . . . been in trouble with the principal for having become 'too involved' with a family, as it was euphemistically put. All I had tried to do was to relate to them in a meaningful way, what I saw to be happening to the patient here in hospital. It seems that we can go and chat with relatives, be supportive, and assure them that all's well with the patient, but we cannot go beyond that (3504).

It was noted in the earlier summary of the dissident ideology that those staff who subscribed to it, tended to be most aware of power differences between themselves and the psychiatrists. It was also they who were most open about their awareness of being direct.

However, the much more striking phenomena was the most general denial of immediate control or direction. If this is taken as reflecting the reality of the situation as experienced by lay staff, then the significance of this absence of direction must be noted. For, if we recall the way nearly all the psychiatrists stressed their 'leadership' role and the way they felt it was up to them to decide the relevance of the lay staff's contribution then the absence of renewed direction would seem to suggest that most lay staff work in such a way that the psychiatrists have no cause to direct them.

Discussion

In the analysis of the first category of ideology, namely that of the welfare workers and testers, attention was drawn to the way that these staff defined themselves as auxiliaries, while the professionals and therapists liked to think of themselves as having a complementary relationship with the psychiatrists. Many of the 'professional' psychologists appeared to be in something of a dilemma over this. For they so qualified the nature of their relationship with the psychiatrists, that they often characterised themselves as being like 'auxiliaries', while stating that they ought to have a complementary relationship with them. The heuristic value of the ideologies can thus be demonstrated when considering the different ways that staff represented the social structure. Within these ideologies, it was suggested that there was a series of interlocking beliefs, assumptions and values about the relevance of their own contribution and that of the other staff, the nature of the division of labour, the legitimacy of the psychiatrists' authority and so on. It is believed that the compatibility of the lay staff's actions with the psychiatrists' expectations can, to a certain extent, be accounted for by the way all these ideologies, with the exception of the dissident one, stressed the need to be 'realistic' in accepting the psychiatrists' 'legal' responsibility.

Nearly all the staff noted how rarely they disagreed with the psychiatrists over matters to do with patients. This suggests an underlying consensus, not only over the question of who does what, but over the structure and functions of the mental health services. Of course many criticisms were levelled against the 'inadequacies' of the present services, even if many also expressed a sense of hopelessness or fatalism about changing things. In this way many lay staff imbued their working relationships with a certain facticity. A consequence of this reification was the perception of working arrangements as being 'natural', 'appropriate' or 'inevitable'. Subjectively many lay staff felt there was little direction over them, although objectively this may have been the case. But this does not necessarily mean that they had autonomy in their actions, other than in those which fell within the boundaries that had been established by themselves or by their own superiors, who were themselves acting on their intepretations of the psychiatrists' expectations. The way that they may have imposed boundaries around their work after experiencing disapproval, or in anticipation of it, is an interesting example of the way control and stability are often maintained within institutions that seek to win the moral involvement of their members.

The fact that there were also staff who were conscious of being directed, suggests that there were not only differences in working relationships, but also different expectations for both self and other within these relationships. So many qualifications were expressed by the lay staff about their relationships with psychiatrists, that it would be a mistake to suggest that it was only the dissidents who felt themselves to be constrained. However, they were the most forthright in saying where they thought they were constrained, and it was they who located the basis of their problems in the psychiatrists' authority, rather than in the personalities or levels of maturity of themselves or the psychiatrists.

Conclusions

This paper has only dealt with certain aspects of the material collected during the study. However, it is believed the questions that have been discussed are central to developing an understanding of the process of professionalisation that goes beyond merely identifying characteristics or stages to consider the nature of the control and autonomy enjoyed by 'emerging' professions. Any occupation can claim to be a profession, but it is only those that are able to control the terms on which they work that are likely to gain the status and regard that are believed to go along with professional recognition. It has only been possible to refer briefly to the varied ways in which the social workers and psychologists viewed the 'professionalisation' of their occupations. While some were in favour, as many were apathetic if not hostile to this issue. When taken alongside the quite different expertise and mandates that were being claimed within the ideologies, it becomes apparent that while associational developments may create the appearance of unity and greater professional assertiveness, at the level of the individual practitioner we are more likely to see accommodation to the *status quo* and an endeavour to gain acceptance from particular psychiatrists. The lay staff enter a situation in which they frequently have considerable freedom in so far as no one is likely to tell them what to do. However, while many lay staff remain critical of the psychiatrists for their inadequate training and reliance on physical methods, they continually reaffirm their authority through a process of defining themselves out of certain areas of work and seeking to involve themselves in various marginal activities.

In terms of their control over resources, procedures and facilities, the lay staff remain in an 'objectively' inferior position to that of the psychiatrists. They may have free access to patients and be able to practice certain kinds of therapy, but such recognition is generally only afforded by particular psychiatrists and is dependent on them sharing the same assumptions about both the nature of mental illness and the reciprocal roles of the occupations involved. Such complementarity, when it occurs, should be considered to be remarkable, bearing in mind the wider lack of agreement over the causes and treatment of mental illness.

This paper also draws attention to certain general problems when considering the social structure of 'team work', and other situations where there is an accent on participation and equality, yet where disparities in power remain. In such situations, stability is maintained as much through the way the subordinates define themselves as having an inferior role to play, as by the superordinates' use of their authority. The occasional use of this authority serves as a reminder of the ultimate differences between them. However, while the division of labour may have been imposed by psychiatrists, it continues to be maintained by the very staff who occupy an inferior position within it.

Notes

1. Ben-David (1963) and Moore (1970) both list nearly 700 references each.
2. See for example Elliott (1972) and Johnson (1972). Johnson's criticisms of earlier theories influenced the approach taken in this paper.
3. Professions, whatever else they may be, are still occupations, and thus the latter term is sometimes used in this paper in a generic sense.
4. Marx (1969) has provided an overview of many of these studies. They have also been critically reviewed by Goldie (1974a), chap. 3.
5. The term 'institutional imperative' is taken from Hearn (1968).
6. The best known American studies being those by Strauss *et al.* (1964) and Rushings (1964). These and the many others have been discussed by Goldie (1974a).
7. See for example Dinitz (1959) or Rushings (1964).
8. As described by Goode (1960) and Smith (1952).
9. Glaser (1963) has provided a useful account of the role of such structures.
10. The study by Henry *et al.* (1971) analyses this issue in some detail.
11. Goldie (1976).
12. Goldie (1974b).
13. The situation of the clinical psychologists has been dealt with by Goldie (1975).
14. As expressed by Gill and Horobin (1972).
15. Apart from such studies as that by Sudnow (1967) there is the more recent

work by Bloor (1976) and West (1976).

16. Strauss *et al.* (1964), Bucher and Strauss (1961), Schatzman and Strauss (1963), Bucher and Stelling (1969), Bucher (1969) and Ehrlich and Sabshin (1964).
17. See for example Mills (1940) and more recently Taylor *et al.* (1973).
18. The staff were distributed between nine different treatment settings (seven mental hospitals, a subnormality hospital and a local authority mental health department). At four of these hospitals only psychologists were interviewed. The hospitals were chosen in order to provide certain contrasts, such as that between 'traditional' and 'progressive', while at the same time none were exceptional.
19. It should be stressed that this was a guide and that considerable flexibility had to be used to adapt it to the situation and the particular circumstances of the interviewee. The interviews were recorded in full by hand and then subsequently typed out.
20. For example, several psychiatrists insisted on associating the researcher with social workers as if sociology and social work were the same thing. Further, in so far as periods of non-participant observation were undertaken, many of the problems associated with this activity were encountered.
21. These are dealt with in considerable detail in Goldie (1974a).
22. Goldie (1976).
23. The first numeral of these code numbers indicates the occupation of the interviewee (thus 1 are psychiatrists, 2 psychologists, and 3 social workers). The second number refers to the setting and the last two numerals identify the individual interviewee.
24. The main problems appeared to be at Oakdene where the psychologists were denied access to the medical records. This difficulty did not occur elsewhere.
25. As with other matters, the psychologists would tend to relate their difficulties to their experiences with individual psychiatrists. Various strategies were described to be used when 'uninformed' junior doctors made 'inappropriate' requests. Also in several of the settings the psychologists had developed their own referral form requesting that the psychiatrists state the nature of the problem, without letting them specify the test to be used. For more details on this, see Goldie (1974a).

References

Ben-David, J. (1963). 'Professions in the Class System of Present Day Societies', *Current Sociology,* vol. 12, no. 3, pp. 249-51.

Bloor, M. (1976). 'Professional autonomy and client exclusion: a study in ENT clinics', in Robinson D. and Wadsworth, M. *Studies in Everyday Medical Life.* London, Martin Robertson.

Bucher, R. (1969). 'A Situational Model of Professional Socialisation', unpublished.

Bucher, R. and J. Stelling. (1969). 'Characteristics of Professional Organisation', *Journal of Health and Social Behaviour,* vol. 10, no. 1, pp. 3-15.

Bucher, R. and A. Strauss. (1961). 'Professions in Process', *American Journal of Sociology,* vol. 66, no. 4, pp. 325-34.

Dinitz, S. *et al.* (1959), 'Status Perceptions in a Mental Hospital', *Social Forces,* vol. 38, no. 2, pp. 124-8.
Elliott, P. (1972). *The Sociology of the Professions.* London, Macmillan.
Ehrlich, D. and M. Sabshin. (1964). 'A Study of Sociotherapeutically Orientated Psychiatrists', *Am. J. Orthopsychiatry,* vol. 34, no. 3.
Freidson, E. (ed.). (1963). *The Hospital in Modern Society.* London, Collier-Macmillan.
Freidson, E. (1970). *The Profession of Medicine.* Dodd Mead and Co.
Freidson, E. (1971). *Professional Dominance.* Atherton.
Gill, D. and G. Horobin. (1972). 'Doctors, Patients and the State: Relationships and Decision Making', *Sociological Review,* vol. 20, no. 4, pp. 505-20.
Glaser, W. (1963). 'American and Foreign Hospitals', in Freidson (1963).
Goldie, N. (1974a). 'Professional Processes Among Three Occupational Groups Within The Mental Health Field', unpublished PhD thesis, the City University.
Goldie, N. (1974b).'"Eclecticism" as the Dominant Ideology and its Contribution Towards the Maintenance of the Status Quo in British Psychiatry'. Paper read at National Deviancy Conference on Medical Ideologies at Bath University in September 1974.
Goldie, N. (1975). 'Clinical Psychology: Statutory Lackey or Unwilling and Informal Handmaiden of Psychiatry'. Paper read at British Sociological Association Medical Sociology Conference in November 1975, at York.
Goldie, N. (1976). 'Psychiatry and the Medical Mandate' in D. Robinson and M. Wadsworth, *Studies in Everyday Medical Life,* London, Martin Robertson.
Goode, W.J. (1960). 'Encroachment, Charlatanism, and the Emerging Professions', *Am. Soc. Review,* vol. 25, no. 6, pp. 902-14.
Hearn, H.L. (1968). 'Identity and Institutional Imperatives: The Socialisation of Student Actresses', *Sociological Quarterly,* vol. 9, pp. 47-63.
Henry, W. *et al.* (1971). *The Fifth Profession* San Francisco, Jossey-Bass.
Johnson, T.J. (1972). *Professions and Power.* London, Macmillan.
Marx,J. (1969). 'A Multidimensional Conception of Ideologies in Professional Arenas', *The Pacific Sociological Review,* vol. 12, no. 2, pp. 75-85.
Mills, C.W. (1940). 'The Professional Ideology of Social Pathologists', *Am. J. of Sociology,* vol. 49, Oct. pp. 165-80.
Moore, W.E. (1970). *The Professions: Roles and Rules.* Russell Sage Foundation, New York.
Rushings, W. (1964). *The Psychiatric Professions.* Chapel Hill. University of North Carolina Press.
Schatzman, L. and A. Strauss (1963). 'A Sociology of Psychiatry: A Perspective and Some Organising Foci', *Social Problems,* vol. 14, no. 1, pp. 3-16.
Smith, H.L. (1952). 'Psychiatry: A Social Institution in Process', *Social Forces,* vol. 33, no. 4, pp. 310-16.
Smith H.L. (1955). 'Two Lines of Authority are One Too Many', *Modern Hospitals,* March.
Strauss, A.L. *et al.* (1964). *Psychiatric Ideologies and Institutions.* New York, Free Press.
Sudnow, D. (1967). *Passing On: The Social Organisation of Dying.* Englewood Cliffs, N.J. Prentice Hall.
Taylor, I. *et al.* (1973). *The New Criminology.* London, Routledge, Kegan and Paul.
West, P. (1976). 'The Physical and the Management of Childhood Epilepsy', in D. Robinson and M. Wadsworth, *Studies in Everyday Medical Life.* London, Martin Robertson.

As a field of enquiry, the sociological study of nursing has tended to shadow the sociological study of the medical profession, reproducing the principal themes of the latter in an essentially imitative fashion. This is not to say that it has always been inferior, since the added opportunities for reflection have often led to marked improvements in theoretical and methodological sophistication, as one may observe by contrasting the work of Davis, Olesen and Whittaker on Californian nursing students with that of Becker and his associates on the Kansas medical school. The development of an historical sociology of nursing, however, has lagged in this country. This may reflect the scope of Abel-Smith's achievement in his narrative history of British nursing. With the passage of time, however, others working in the field have begun to chip away at this account. In particular, as Carpenter implies, its excessive concentration on a metropolitan-oriented leadership led to inadequate attention being given to the historical and intellectual movements which underlay the development of general nursing and its gradual takeover of several other discrete occupations – asylum attendants, midwives, health visitors.

The possibility of such an analysis is opened to Carpenter by the shift in perspective exemplified by several other papers in this volume, with its new concentration on hospitals as places of work. Medicine and medical care form a body of tasks whose delineation and distribution are a matter of everyday concern and everyday bargaining at the 'shop floor' of patient contact. The activities of each and every one of the several groups of workers involved become critical subjects for the sociology of medicine. In this instance, we are directed towards an examination of the evolving situation of rank-and-file nursing. We can see how a distinctive area of work was carved, by the abdication of therapy and management as central interests of doctors, to offer a socially acceptable niche for Victorian spinsters. The resulting occupational pattern with its particular style of élite legitimation by ordeal held sway until comparatively recently.

The twin influences of social and technical change have, however, now led to its gradual disintegration. The extension of capitalist rationality to the health service has replaced a moral with a formal basis for élite legitimation. The interests of nursing leaders and the rank and file have increasingly diverged into a classical scheme of management and worker. Carpenter argues that the nursing links of nurse managers are becoming attenuated to the point of possible disappearance for all practical purposes. They are managers first and nurses second. The response of the rank and file is predictable, namely increasing unionisation.

Apart from the issues of nursing policy raised by Carpenter's paper, there are also important sociological implications. Our historical studies have paid too little attention to the rank and file situation in contrast to that of occupational leaders. Similarly, we are still only paying lip-service to a comprehensive study of the division of medical labour. This volume concentrates overwhelmingly on doctors and, to a lesser degree, nurses and social workers. We have included little on the paramedical professions because little work is being done on them and Manson's account, which follows Carpenter's, is one of the few to address the position and actions of ancillary workers. Carpenter shows that work on the range of occupations and professions in the medical division of labour is not only possible but also urgent as we are faced with the need to spell out the implications of applying capitalist reasoning to the nation's health.

R.D.

THE NEW MANAGERIALISM AND PROFESSIONALISM IN NURSING

Michael Carpenter

Introduction

This paper discusses some significant contemporary developments in British nursing, set against an historical background. Although an outstanding historical survey exists,[1] that work is now some years old and, contains little theory on the development of nursing. Occupational politics in the context of changes in occupational content needs emphasising and the familiar picture of an occupation almost totally resistant to change requires considerable modification.

At present there is accelerating change in the NHS, in nursing itself and in society as a whole. It cannot be overemphasised, therefore, that the conclusions and predictions based on contemporary developments are provisional.

The Creation of an Occupational Community

It is a commonplace in labour economics that the provision of occupational services depends on the intersection of the forces of demand and supply. The emergence of nursing at the end of the nineteenth century in the voluntary hospitals is almost a textbook example, just as the later loss of impetus in nursing reform was in many ways due to these forces coming into more or less permanent disequilibrium.

On the supply side, the story has often been narrated of substantial numbers of unmarriageable middle- and upper-middle-class women becoming a burden to their parents. Victorian England was characterised by contradictory developments. On the one hand there was the romantic celebration of the nobility of 'womanhood'. This had many precedents, but it was encouraged by the development among the bourgeoisie of the idea of the 'family' as a 'refuge', to which they could escape at least temporarily from the competitive baseness of the world of Capital. At the same time, there were the first stirrings of women's consciousness, as these women saw a life spread before them without any real social functions.

Nursing emerged as a compromise. Although some leading individuals were involved in the feminist movement, the main thrust of nursing reform was largely congruent with the prevailing male definitions of womanhood. Nursing enabled the desire for some measure of self-determination to be realised in terms agreeable to the prevailing male imagery of women. The work itself was not to be tainted with the world of Capital. It was to be carried out as a *service* and pecuniary motives were to play no part, just as the home was supposed to be the place where goods and services were provided for love, not money. But work in hospitals exposed women to intimate contact with male patients, and put them in close proximity to male doctors. The cloistered separateness of the nursing community served to reassure anxious fathers and was probably decisive in many cases in them allowing their daughters to leave home and take up nursing. The espousal of religious virtues helped to protect the nurse during intimate contact with male patients. The class distance between these women and the majority of their patients, and the ban on 'familiarity' were reinforcing factors. The rigid discipline and the seclusion in the nurses' home, were also part of a network of devices which served to protect the fragile notions of womanhood from the world at large and, more particularly, from doctors. Increasing numbers of these women exchanged one rigidly authoritarian environment for another, compensated by some promise of social worth.

This occupational infrastructure helped to change the existing image of the nurse from a generally disreputable character to that of a ministering angel. It helped to make available a sufficient supply of ladies (and aspiring ladies) for nurse training in the voluntary hospitals. Clearly, however, 'demand' factors were equally important. Nursing reform depended not only on there being work which was either not being done or not being done adequately, but also on the resources nursing leaders could deploy against opponents. In the voluntary hospitals these conditions were more or less met, resulting in the intersection of the forces of demand and supply.

A vacant occupational space occurred initially because reformers could claim that the somewhat diverse elements which were to make up the new occupation (delegated treatments from doctors, care of patients' physical needs, the maintenance of the ward in a clean and proper condition, and so on) could be viewed as a unified whole, in terms of the 'sanitary idea'. This idea emerged before, but was systematised scientifically by the acceptance of the germ theory of disease, which was an important ideal of social reform generally in the nineteenth century. The theory meant that the health of the working class could no longer be ignored by the higher orders, for infective disease was not a 'respector of persons'. As Celia Davies has pointed out, the sanitary idea formed the knowledge basis of early nursing.[2]

The emphasis on 'hygiene' had a number of important consequences for the claim to occupational recognition. It meant first that 'the proper duties of the nurse' straddled both the scientific and the non-scientific worlds. The vocational idea that care of the sick and attention to their needs was noble in itself was certainly present. Just as important was the idea that nurses should either understand the importance of hygiene in carrying out all their various menial and less menial duties, or that those who did understand should control those who carried them out. At the outset, therefore, nursing tasks were defined less by what they involved, and more by the principles underlying them. Even the scrubbing of floors was partly lit by the glow of medical science. The principles of medical science had to be transmitted to nurses in their training, although deep divisions emerged among nursing leaders on the necessary extent of this training. The implementation of this knowledge required military organisation and regimentation in the battle against disease. It meant controlling rather than indulging patients, in the interests of hygiene.

The beauty of the idea lay in its simplicity, serving in turn to unify the occupation into a single community stretching from the lowest ranking to the highest ranking nurse. The crucial element in the situation was the power of the matron. As Nightingale wrote: 'The whole reform in nursing both at home and abroad has consisted in this; To take all power over the nursing out of the hands of the men, and put it into the hands of *one female* trained head and make her responsible for everything (regarding internal management and discipline)' (emphasis in the original).[3] The power lodged in the single figure was a means of practical reform. As upper-class women the matrons were able, if required, to go above the heads of stewards, and sometimes even doctors, to influence social peers on the Boards of Governors and beyond. They used their powers to bring to heel or if necessary replace (under the banner of the sanitary idea) the existing nursing staff and domestics on the wards. At the same time they recognised the importance of obedience in clinical matters to the doctors, while asserting partial autonomy by insisting that physicians could not themselves directly discipline nurses.

At this time doctors were becoming increasingly interested in the diagnostic aspects of illness rather than treatment, and were thus prepared to allow some functions to be delegated under their control. They were little interested in and ill-equipped by their training to deal with matters of ward and hospital administration. Then, as now, their focus was largely upon symptoms. The emergence of a new occupation which was prepared humbly to carry out clinical and administrative tasks offered great advantages for doctors.

What emerged was the reproduction of the Victorian class structure in the hospital, based on the division of labour between the sexes, and between women of different classes. With the initial advances in medical science and the new forms of social organisation which developed in voluntary hospitals at the end of the nineteenth century, the idea took root that the process of 'cure' was separate from and superior to that of 'care'. Sex, class and later racial insignia were attached to this division as the basis for hospital stratification. Cure functions were seen as primarily male and upper class, and care functions predominantly lower class and/or female but, initially at least, carried out under the moral leadership of upper-class women. The social position occupied by the matron in the hospital power structure, involving the supervision of the majority of aspects of the care structure, bore a close relation to the position she might have occupied, as an upper-middle-class woman in the Victorian home, had she married. In claiming supreme authority over all female staff there was the precedent of the lady of the house, whose supervision of servants complemented but did not subvert the authority of her husband.[4]

Thus towards the end of the nineteenth century the term 'matron' took on a new and additional meaning. Previously it had meant powers exercised in an institution by virtue of being the wife of the steward. In the voluntary hospitals, matrons exercised a new power by becoming the symbolic wife of the doctor, and in so doing helped to establish a sphere of autonomy and not just submission. The matron's autonomy lay chiefly in the managerial control of those under her. Over those she ruled there were basically two strands of legitimation. For some there was the promise of career and a future position of rank, either as a matron or ward sister. In the early days promotion was especially rapid for the Lady Pupils who paid for their training, many of whom became matrons almost on completion of training. For those at the base of the care structure, the lower-ranking nurses and maids, the matron must have been legitimated as mistress of the house.

The imagery of nursing was almost perfectly adapted to the power realities of the voluntary hospitals, and the definition of what was nurses' work was sufficiently flexible to expand to fit the available jobs to be done. Yet nursing tasks remained unified because of the sanitary idea. Besides, nursing encompassed a fairly limited range of activities.

The varieties of clinical treatments and drugs were not great in comparison with today, and the managerial abilities required were largely routine. Most of all there was just hard, unremitting work, the basic essentials of which did not vary greatly from one nursing situation to the next. At this time the total body of knowledge required by a nurse was within the capacities of a single intelligent person, which made the matron into a universalistic nursing authority: an educator, administrator and repository of experience, but first of all a nurse. It was on this basis that nurses once trained were able to carry out nursing reforms in any likely setting.

Setbacks and Survival

The many factors which came together in the voluntary hospitals were either absent or only partially present elsewhere. There were considerable obstacles to the kinds of nursing reforms desired by the emergent élite, which had established itself in the voluntary hospitals. In this paper two selective examples are followed through: the workhouse hospitals and the asylums. A more thorough historical account would cover other areas more extensively. The obstacles were of two kinds: an often radically different balance of power in other settings, combined with changing circumstances in society as a whole.

The most important of the latter forces lay in the fact that the voluntary hospital élite were pressing the state for some kind of professional autonomy, although divided among themselves to some extent, at the same time that the state was assuming greater responsibility for health care, a process considerably hastened by the First World War. Many nurses had to be found and trained quickly during the war. They were admitted in large numbers as Voluntary Aid Detachments (VADs), many of whom posed problems of assimilation to the register of nurses, finally established after the war, and considerable professional pressure was exerted against such 'dilutees'. This issue was not resolved finally until the newly-formed Ministry of Health enforced the rights of VADs and others to be admitted to the register. Neither should it be overlooked that this also took place at a time of swingeing cuts in public expenditure in the 1920s. The claim for some kind of autonomy was trapped in the contradiction that the state was assuming greater responsibility for health care at the same time that it was cutting back on its cost. This was an unfortunate conjuncture of circumstances for the occupational élite.

Many of the wider social forces were more localised in effect, however. Towards the end of the nineteenth century pauperism and ill health began to be distinguished and the inappropriateness of the doctrines of 'less-eligibility' for dealing with the sick, the old and the insane were slowly acknowledged. Yet in the absence of any massive central funding, which did not really occur until 1948, reform was resisted locally by the middle class concerned at the rise in the poor rate. This was compounded by the long years of recession in the last decades of the nineteenth century.

In addition to these difficulties, nurse reformers in workhouse hospitals found less of a vacant occupational space then they had in the voluntary hospitals. There was an established professional management of a sort: the workhouse masters. In addition medical officers more often combined administrative and clinical duties. Even the preparedness of Nightingale nurses to work for low wages could scarcely compete with the even more inexpensive pauper nurse. In any case, workhouse masters often preferred pauper nurses because they could be more easily controlled than trained nurses. Well into the twentieth century masters rather than matrons were in control of nurses. In fact, under the poor law regulations they were called Nursing Superintendents, indicating their more limited role.[4]

The situation in the asylums was a little different, and the élite experienced some success. During the early 1900s, often with the connivance of psychiatrists, Nightingale-trained nurses were brought in as assistant matrons or matrons. A full account and explanation of these events must wait detailed historical research. However, it seems that two factors were of great significance. At around this time the medical model of psychiatric disorder was beginning its ascendancy. Further, women nurses were being brought in to implement newer methods of treatment based less on physical coercion, even though it is now apparent that the Nightingale nurses brought their inappropriate bureaucratic rigidities with them, in what has been called the 'hospitalisation' of the asylums.

This was an early example of a trend of some importance in the development of twentieth-century nursing. The original adaptability of nursing was nevertheless unified under the sanitary idea. Nursing gradually assimilated many diverse sets of responsibilities that had increasingly little connection with the original sanitary idea. This has, cumulatively, led to a crisis of occupational identity, which is discussed later.

The hospitalisation of the asylums was encouraged by psychiatrists, but the nursing élite also showed enthusiasm rather than merely obeisance. Indeed, this development (as well as the attempted reforms of workhouse nursing), can be seen as analogous to wider social events. It was part of a nursing 'imperialism' whereby the élite of the voluntary hospitals attempted to extend its influence and subordinate other occupations defined as inferior in terms of status to the 'metropolitan' occupation, general nursing in the voluntary hospitals.

The existing male attendants were badly placed to fend off this attempted take-over. They were generally of a much lower class than the matrons and, at the time, had little independent awareness of their occupational status or desire to advance it. Thus the initiatives for training schemes and pressures towards professionalisation emanated in the main from psychiatrists, who may have seen it partly as a way of advancing their own occupational status. When attendants began to articulate an independent identity it was, initially at least, largely preoccupied with *compensatory* aspects of doing an unpleasant job, in particular focusing on pensions, pay, hours and discipline.[5] In these circumstances women nurses could and were used to undercut male attendants. The union, the National Asylum Workers' Union, was one of the first in Britain to pursue a policy of equal pay, partly as a strategy for making it unattractive for management to hire female labour.[6] Nevertheless, before the development of psychotropic drugs, male attendants had a guaranteed place for the social control of patients. They also fought against coming under the direct authority of women, and restricted the powers of matrons largely to the female wards. However, during the First World War, when large numbers of male attendants enlisted in the forces, women nurses were increasingly employed on male sides, thus extending the matrons' authority. The position of male psychiatric nurses further declined as a result of the 1919 Nurses Act. The legislation set up a separate male register and barred them from the general register, thus making advancement virtually impossible and severely restricting their mobility.

Adaptability and readiness to absorb changes in job content, was matched by a profound conservatism in the occupational infrastructure (i.e. the social organisation of nursing as an occupation). Most authors see this conservatism as responsible for increasing problems of nursing shortages, despite substantial increases in the numbers of nurses. These increases could not cope with demand. Abel-Smith suggests that the problem was a shortage of all types of nurses.[7] The occupational élite made some concessions in the inter-war period, by admitting recruits at a lower age, by some reduction of hours and improvement of pay, though, significantly, most of these concessions occurred outside the voluntary hospitals. On one point they were extremely reluctant to compromise, namely the idea that nursing should be a life-long vocation. This in turn necessitated the continuation of both a cloistered life and a harsh authoritarian régime. The matron élite, so flexible on many issues, exhibited considerable rigidity when it came to changing the infrastructure.

It still has not been satisfactorily explained why this strategy survived so long after it appeared to most outsiders to be anachronistic. A clue is given in a statement made by a member of the élite in 1916, that 'It is questionable if the best type of women ever resents reasonable authority. Experience teaches that a probationer who objects to authority is an unsuitable candidate for the nursing profession, and will make trouble if kept.'[8] The élite demanded that nursing took priority in all spheres of life, work and non-work. This insistence acted both as a deterrent to recruitment of many potentially good nurses, and served to expel those who either could or would not give total commitment.

At this time, as from the onset, nursing was bureaucratically organised. This bureaucratic organisation (perhaps autocratic would be a better word) should not be seen as in any real way analagous to the later development of 'managerialism' in nursing. To borrow from Max Weber, it was a strategy based on *Wertrationalität,* the single minded pursuit of an absolute value, rather than on *Zweckrationalität* whereby, as in capitalist economic rationality, action is based on the 'rational' weighing of alternatives in the light of their utility. In other words, the conservative infrastructure was designed more to help achieve and maintain an occupational community than to make best available use of labour resources. Low pay and the requirement of living-in would, it was hoped, ensure that only suitable inspired neophytes were recruited. Continuing inflexibility, harsh conditions and long hours enabled the élite to discover and eject those who escaped the initial net and could not maintain their levels of commitment. At each stage of career advancement these demands increased. It was very wasteful of highly-skilled nurses who, for example, would leave when they married. It ensured, however, that only those with the highest levels of motivation reached the apex of the occupation, guaranteeing the survival and transmission of the occupational ideals from one generation to the next.

The hostility to male nurses noted by Abel-Smith[9] may have been partly due to the factors he mentions, and also to a feeling on the part of the elite that male nurses might threaten this delicate structure of harsh discipline, total commitment and low pay. For male nurses did not share any of these values, but nevertheless saw nursing as a life-long occupation. The danger was that they might introduce a very different rationality if they ever achieved positions of influence. This may have been an important reason for the exclusion from general nursing of males, whose rather different orientations to work were observed at close hand in the mental hospitals.

The wasteful personnel policies served the élite's interests in other ways. Given a pyramidal structure, they limited the number of career nurses who were chasing the few posts at the top. The voluntary hospitals were also able to export many of their career-minded graduates to positions of high rank in the other nursing services. This was in turn made possible by the other sectors, like poor law facilities and asylums, employing larger numbers of lower-class, less career-minded recruits. In these sectors nursing was more often carried out by women with few alternative employment opportunities, who either tolerated the conditions as a stop gap between school and marriage; or for whom, as single women on a permanent basis, living-in provided perhaps a security they might not have otherwise enjoyed. All these complex elements fitted together, not necessarily as a conscious conspiracy, in ways which enabled the infrastructure to survive for many years, but which did not favour the full realisation of a stable occupational community.

An Occupational Community in Crisis

By the end of the 1950s, there was disequilibrium in the delicate balance of forces which had maintained the occupational infrastructure for so long. Perhaps the most important factor was the assumption by the state of the major responsibility for health care. This process had begun during the Second World War, and the most immediate effect was the raising of student nurses' salaries against the vigorous opposition of the Royal College of Nursing (Rcn). The next step, the Nurses Act 1943, represented a compromise in favour of the occupational élite. A second grade of assistant nurse with shortened training was introduced. She was to have no prospect of career advancement and would pose no threat of dilution to registered nurses. Not surprisingly, this grade was not a great success and after the war shortages increasingly became apparent. The creation of the National Health Service (NHS) meant that some new compromise had to be found. Criteria of economic rationality began to be applied. The resistance to male, married and part-time nurses was less tenable. The élite were forced to admit more untrained orderlies and aides, but as Abel-Smith notes:

> The leaders of the nursing profession were not, however, willing to sanction the performance of basic nursing duties by these grades. They intended that all such work would be reserved for registered

nurses, assistant nurses, and those in training for these grades.[10]

A major reason for the maturation of the crisis in the 1960s was the ineffectiveness of this compromise in the light of the profound changes in job content which had taken place. These changes affected nursing in hospital most where health care was increasingly concentrated and where nursing took an increasing part of the health budget. The changes in job content were mainly of three types. First, an increasing number of clinical responsibilities were being delegated, as a result of the growth of scientific medicine. Second, there had been an increase in the importance of the nurse as a coordinator of a wide number of ancillary functions in the ward or department. These functions had expanded primarily as a result of the development of large and complex institutions, and the emergence of 'paramedical' occupations and departments with only intermittent contact with patients.[11] The third type followed partly from the scientific developments, which have paradoxically increased the numbers of chronically ill and infirm patients who require long-term routine care. This, perhaps more than anything, has changed the nature of nursing work.

In contrast to the past, when the range of nursing tasks was relatively limited and unified, they were now so varied that the temptation was to begin to stratify activities along these three main divides. While training was seen as necessary in the light of changes in the first two types of activities, this did not necessarily apply to the third to any great extent. As Abel-Smith shows, at the onset of the NHS, nurses were still reluctant to hand over basic nursing duties to auxiliaries. As the proportion of chronically sick patients increased, the job satisfaction in carrying out basic nursing tasks declined. The nursing élite began to look more towards the clinical and managerial aspects of their work. Their desire to offload 'dirty' or routine work onto other groups under their control, could be articulated in terms of economic rationality, namely the economic use of trained labour. This meant an increasing abandonment of traditional nursing values, as basic nursing was devolved to untrained nursing auxiliaries.

As at other times in the development of nursing, there was a conjuncture of circumstances. The NHS had seen considerable investment in hospital building and more was promised under the Hospital Plan of 1962. The assistant nurse grade had not been successful in attracting larger numbers to basic nursing as it had no career ladder. And, for a complex set of reasons, training for the register was not attracting sufficient numbers of middle-class girls.

They now had other outlets which did not require of them single-minded commitment. For example, a survey of 302 'intelligent' schoolgirls in Yorkshire in 1964 showed that 67 per cent expressed no interest in nursing.[12] Increasing resort was made to overseas nurses, whose mobility out of nursing were severely restricted because of the problem of work permits. Nursing management was still based largely on the authority of the matron. There was a chronic shortage of applicants for nursing administration posts.[13]

The New Managerialism

The particular balance of forces at the beginning of the 1960s gave emphasis to the managerial rather than the clinical changes in job content. The élite were particularly concerned with the declining status of nurse managers in comparison to other occupational groups, especially in the teaching hospitals. As the Salmon Report on Nursing Management noted in 1966:

> While the status of matrons in former local authority hospitals generally improved, in many voluntary hospitals it declined. The intimate relation of the matron with Governors who were concerned with a single hospital could not be maintained in a group of hospitals, perhaps fifteen or more each with its own Matron with access in some groups only to a House Committee. In some groups the position of Matron compared unfavourably with that of the Group Secretary and of the medical staff, whose influence was exercised at the level of the governing body.[14]

Although policy throughout the 1950s had been that nurse managers should have access to all relevant committees, the conditions were not always met.

The large district general hospital proposed in the 1962 plan provided the most explicit basis for the alliance between the occupational élite and the state for a managerial solution. The view of the Salmon Committee on the hospital plan was that technological hardware is 'usually expensive and expert management will be needed, in which nurses should play their part, if costs are to be held in check'.[15] The state sought manageable labour costs in the use of nurses and ancillary workers. Nurses, however, were affected in more oblique ways. Tasks which could be practically and aesthetically subjected to productivity criteria (such as those based on work study techniques) were hived off to lay management. No bonus schemes were introduced for nurses, but there were attempts to minimise wage costs by other means. First, as Manson shows, in another paper in this volume,[16] there were pressures to divide skilled and unskilled elements of nursing work. Second, more progressive personnel policies were implemented to enable a fuller exploitation of an available labour force. In contrast to traditional values, these meant increasing the number of part-time and married women in the labour force, in jobs with little career opportunities. It also led the National Board for Prices and Incomes (NBPI) in their Report No. 60, to recommend the ending of petty restrictions and interference in the personal lives of student nurses living in homes. This had an explicit economic rationale. The report did not believe that big increases in student nurses' pay were necessary for 'the problem is more one of retention than recruitment, and retention can be helped by means other than a general pay increase.'[17] Indeed, the increasing popularity of the term 'wastage' in élite circles at this time, is highly indicative of a new managerial approach to labour resources. A more participative style of management might help increase job satisfaction at ward level and lessen nurses' tendency to leave, especially since local managers were unable, given the highly centralised machinery for wage and salary determination, to raise the wages of nurses. By creating a new image for nursing and flexibility on the part of management, trained staff could be attracted back. Further, the élite wanted to create a 'career' structure that might entice back some of the middle-class recruits. Above all the strategic position of nursing in the hospital division of labour and its importance for the continuity of care, made it imperative to plan the utilisation of labour resources.

Thus the desire of élite elements to restore some of their lost influence and increase the status of nursing as an occupation, coincided with the state's desire for greater efficiency in the use of labour. It was necessary, however, for the élite to engage in a thorough self-criticism of their traditions. This occurred when the nursing élite, who formed the sole nursing voice on the Salmon Committee,[18] participated with managerial experts in a savage attack upon the matron system of management. The tenor of the resulting report is two-fold. First, traditional nursing and modern business administration are contrasted and the former pronounced inferior to the latter. Second, the established methods of business administration are said to form a separate body of knowledge, managerial science, which are entirely suitable to nursing, as they are to any other form of administration. Thus the report states:

> In nursing administration effective delegation is rarely seen . . . the Matron of a sizeable hospital may head an array of deputy assistants and administrative sisters to whom she assigns duties, *but she does not find the relief that the top person of a business seems to find.* She often retains work that she could well hand over to assistants.[19]

Salmon implicitly called for a managerial structure based on the industrial model of professionalised management as under advanced monopoly capitalism, where a corps of professional managers have tended to replace individual owner entrepreneurs. This structure includes a growing army of middle management. The Matron system of managerialism is almost an archetypal system of unitary management[20] that, though quite adaptable to small and less complex institutions was inappropriate for the larger hospitals that official thinking now favoured. 'The job of a Matron of a 1,000 bedded General Hospital and of the Matron of a Cottage Hospital of say, 30 beds should have about as much in common *as those of a Sales Director of a fair sized manufacturing firm and the manager of a small business*.'[21] A different form of bureaucracy based on a fundamentally new kind of rationality was advocated by Salmon.[22] Its essence was that the managerial chain was lengthened both above and below the matron, both to meet the demands by matrons for influence at group level, and also in the hope of creating a career structure which would enable nursing to compete again with other middle-class occupations. The new structure is summarised in Figure 1.

Figure 1 The Salmon System of Nursing Management

Grade	Title	Sphere of Authority	Formerly for example
10	Chief Nursing Officer (CNO)	Group	–
9	Principal Nursing Officer (PNO)	Division	Large Hospital
8	Senior Nursing Officer (SNO)	Area	Medium-Sized Hospital
7	Nursing Officer (NO)	Unit	Small Hospital/ Group of Wards
6	Sister/Charge Nurse	Section	Ward
5	Staff Nurse	Section	Ward

Nurses were to be relieved of direct control of what were called 'non-nursing' services which had often been carried out from the early days of nursing reform. Now nurses had absorbed many more complex managerial functions and the élite wished to relieve themselves of these routine tasks.[23] There was an alliance between members of the élite, who found the routine tasks tiresome, and the state wishing to economise on skilled manpower and subject such jobs to productivity criteria. Once freed from these onerous tasks, the élite would be better placed to engage in higher planning functions and move closer towards parity with other élite groups.

The Impact of the New Managerialism

The occupational élite had seen in the proposals of the Salmon Report a way of renewing themselves and for that reason had been prepared to abandon tradition. This was bound to threaten the already fragile occupational community and create new rifts. Three main and interconnected sets of factors must be considered: first, the effect of the new nursing managerialism on other occupational groups, primarily in the hospital superstructure; second, the effect on the managers themselves; third, the effect upon more subordinated nurses.

Medical interests were unusually absent in formulating the Salmon changes. There was only one physician member of the Salmon Committee yet Salmon created a potential for greater control by nurses in clinical matters. This has been reflected in particular by the ways in which some nursing officers have interpreted their job, and not surprisingly they have tended to irritate some consultants.[24] Doctors seem to have woken up rather belatedly to this potential threat.[25] Some nurses apparently experience a sense of anomie (like the nurses who periodically write individually and in groups to the nursing press asking for matrons to be brought back). In addition, ward-level nurses resent the new reward structure which they feel is stacked against them. Ward sisters, much of whose work is managerial (in the sense outlined by Mauksch) may nevertheless often continue to think of themselves in terms of the traditional image of the bedside nurse and scorn 'managers' and what they see as 'useless' committee work.

The defence of those who favour Salmon has tended to be that there is nothing intrinsically wrong with its principles. The problem is rather that nurses fail to understand them and do not work to the spirit of the recommendations. It is argued that many nurse managers either carry on as before or mistakenly interpret the Report as implying an excessively bureaucratic view of managerial functions. As the official report *Progress on Salmon* noted in 1972: 'One of the most pressing problems remains; this is the lack of understanding about what the Salmon

Report actually says.'[26] Not surprisingly this view also coincided with 'advanced' thinking in the profession. Eve Bendall warned, for example, in 1966 that 'while the structure is clear on paper, the inbred attitudes in the profession will make the changeover far from easy'.[27] Was it so clear? The proposals seem to pursue contradictory objectives: towards greater bureaucracy in order to create the career structures to satisfy the aspirations of the occupational élite and towards decentralisation to improve the job satisfaction and retention of ward level staff.

Undoubtedly these problems were exacerbated by the haste with which the proposals were implemented following the publication of the NBPI Report No. 60, without fully testing them in pilot schemes. This generated considerable anxiety amongst existing nurse managers, many of whom were finally assimilated to new positions of responsibility, the demands of which they did not fully understand.[28] Given the particular authoritarian milieu, it is not surprising that the bureaucratic rather than the decentralistising tendencies of Salmon tended so often to get the upper hand. It appears that, not surprisingly, community nurses have tended to resist bureaucratic encroachment most. Their work situation, for reasons suggested by Victor Jupp,[29] is not one which is easily subjected to managerial control. It is also ironically rather more professionalised as community nurses carry out care and 'advise' lay relatives rather than 'supervise' untrained nursing staff who are paid wages.

Haste in implementation left no transition period during which larger numbers of middle-class women could be attracted to nursing as hoped by the élite. The target date set by the NBPI Report No. 60 in March 1968 was for 1 January 1969. As noted earlier, there had been a continuous shortage of numbers applying for administrative posts in the past. Despite appearance to the contrary, it seems untrue that Salmon greatly expanded the number of available posts.[30] However, despite open competition for posts it seems that large numbers of people with no great ability were rapidly assimilated from old to new positions with little time to prepare them for assuming their new responsibilities.

In this situation male nurses were well placed to compete for positions. As NBPI Report No. 60 noted in the psychiatric field, male nurses 'are older and give longer service than the equivalent grade in General Hospitals. Their promotion prospects are much poorer than those of female nursing staff. Male staff nurses have an average length of service of nearly seven years in that grade, female staff nurses of three years.'[31] Female opportunities in this field were undoubtedly greater. An article in *Nursing Times* in 1963 on 'How to Become a Matron' advised ambitious girls that they could become matrons much more rapidly in psychiatric than general hospitals.[32] Male nurses were generally considered of lower status and confined to male sides. In 1959 Jones's and Sidebotham's case studies found that matrons often controlled training schools and the administrative block, while the influence of chief male nurses was found typically to be 'confined largely to the male block and does not extend to the hospital as a whole'.[33] In contrast to general hospitals there were no shortages of applications for administrative posts in psychiatric hospitals. Yet despite the fact that career 'bottlenecks' existed at ward level, nursing tended, as Robert Dingwall argued, to represent 'upward social mobility, which leads them to emphasise the professional and career aspects of the occupation'.[34] Thus during the 1950s and 60s many male psychiatric nurses sought secondment for postgraduate general training to obtain the SRN thought so necessary for career advancement in any field. Some mental handicap hospitals, for example, had matrons with SRN but no qualification in the subnormality field.[35]

Salmon suddenly provided outlets for long-standing and largely frustrated aspirations. Many male nurses possessed traits which tended to propel them up the new hierarchies: they were more likely to stay longer in the service, to work full-time (part-time status often being a bar to promotion), to wish to escape low pay and perhaps a feeling of marginality in the clinical situation and, perhaps most signficant of all, to have greater geographical mobility than their female competitors. By ending the sex divided structure in particular, Salmon opened up new channels of mobility for men to rise to high administrative positions. Yet there were other, less transparent, reasons why men should suddenly be favoured. Salmon hardly mentioned the role of men, but there is no doubt that in redefining 'female' positions into strictly functional managerial ones they were made ripe for male capture. In the past men, as men, could not be expected to possess the 'qualities' of a good nurse, or if they did, were often considered effeminate and thus less than men. Salmon transformed the image of men in nursing. They are now perceived to possess 'managerial' traits. Their previous disadvantages make them potentially good administrators.

The Salmon Report was an implicit critique of *female* authority and as such is sexist. Female nurses are viewed almost as inherently unable to exercise administrative skills. They may be 'meticulous in details on which the life of a patient depends', which may be admirable qualities for a ward nurse, 'but when, on promotion to posts in Matron's office they venture on to "administration" many seem unable to take decisions'.[36] Men in our society are credited with greater ability to take decisions. They are less open to the charge of trivial and obsessive spinsterhood that seems to lie behind the talk of being 'meticulous in details'. Apart from this, men are considered tougher material for the world of management, or as the *Nursing Times* put it in 1963, 'men may find it easier to stand the physical and nervous strain of the top job than many women do'.[37]

Because of the lower-class origins and less monastic life style of male nurse managers other modern virtues could be ascribed to them. They were less open to the charge of social snobbery and thus capable of dealing with junior staff more sensitively and sympathetically. Usually men from working-class origins are only admitted into the higher echelons of the class structure after a prolonged period of socialisation designed in part to dissolve previous loyalties. Many of the new male nurse managers, however, were suddenly promoted to power, before such a process could take place. They, therefore, might be expected to retain at least initially many of their previous attitudes and dispositions. They might, for example, be more ready to negotiate with and recognise trade unions. Many would remain trade unionists themselves. The new impersonality and larger scale of the management structure would, of course, weaken patronage and encourage the spread of trade unionism, which is as much a feature of the regularisation of personnel policies as an oppositional institution. Whether the new male nurse managers were members of the Rcn as well as, or rather than, members of trade unions they expected that organisation to take much more of a trade union stance than it had in the past. This may help explain partially the increased dynamism of the Rcn in recent years.

All these factors contributed to the dramatic trends noted (but unfortunately not explained) by Brown and Stones in 1972: 'In all types of hospitals the number of men in the top two grades of PNO and CNO increased eightfold between 1969 and 1972 compared to only a fivefold increase for females. In 1972 men occupied a third of all these posts. There was only one female PNO in a mental hospital.'[38] By grasping opportunities for mobility as they appeared, the new male managers were helping to transform social control within hospitals. In the past nurses had tended to be indirectly dominated by men in the medical profession, but the immediate structure of domination has been primarily that of class through upper-middle-class women. These women are now increasingly being replaced by male nurse managers of much more humble origins. It is almost as if the declining potency of class domination of women by women necessitates a much more direct form of sex domination of men over women from *within* nursing.

Reorganisation and After

More recent figures supplied to me for 30 October 1974 by the DHSS suggest that the situation has stabilised since reorganisation. At the DNO/Grade 10 level for all hospitals the proportion of male nurses is approximately 30 per cent. At Divisional Nursing Officer/PNO/Director of Nursing Services level a little lower down the hierarchy it stands somewhat higher at approximately 34 per cent. Towards the higher reaches, at area level, there are fewer male nurses, though at around 20 per cent they occur twice as frequently as in the nursing labour force as a whole. In the mental illness and handicap hospitals there is more male domination – around 70 per cent of all posts above ward sister/charge nurse are occupied by men who comprise about 32 per cent of the labour force. The impression created is that male nurses have scaled all the cliffs at hospital level, but have yet to monopolise the pinnacles in the clouds at area level and beyond. This might be expected given their fairly recent rise to prominence.

The consequences of the reorganisation of the NHS in 1973 in fracturing the occupational community of nursing are almost as great as Salmon itself, when taken with the dramatically changing economic scene. In one sense reorganisation involves a continuation of the same logic by fully integrating nurse management with other forms of management on an equal basis. The PNO and CNO disappear. Above SNO, new positions are called into existence. The Divisional Nursing Officer (DivNO) replaces what was roughly the PNO. He, or she, is now responsible to the District Nursing Officer, who is an equal member of the District Management Team (DMT) and directly accountable to the Area Health Authority (AHA). Similarly, the Area Nursing Officer (ANO) is a member of the Area Team of Officers (ATO) and also accountable to the AHA. The Regional Nursing Officer (RNO) is an equal member of the Regional Team of Officers (RTO) and accountable to the Regional Health Authority (RHA). This complex, bewildering structure is summarised in Figure 2.

Within this new structure nurse managers are supposed to participate as full and equal members of managerial teams which, in deference primarily to medical interests, are 'teams of equals' – consensus bodies where each member has the power of veto. On the DMT, for example, the nurse manager shares this new power with the District Community Physician, the District Administrator, the District Finance Officer, and two elected medical representatives of consultants and general practitioners. Nurse managers have never before possessed so much potential power.

Figure 2 The New Patterns of Nursing Management

Title of 'Role'	Full Member of:	Has Direct Authority over:	'Monitors and Coordinates':	Is Accountable to:
RNO	RTO		ANO	RHA
ANO	ATO		DNO	AHA
DNO	DNT	DivNOs		
DivNO	–	SNOs	–	Rank superior
SNO	–		–	Rank superior

The other notable feature of the structure, as it radiates upwards from SNOs through the Divisional Nursing Officers to the District and above, is that nurse management really begins to appear similar to an economic 'conglomerate'. District Nursing Officers head a managerial empire which involves overseeing not only their own staff but also heading lesser empires beneath them. As there is a single channel of upward mobility from all nursing disciplines, 'disciplinary' background becomes of diminishing importance to career advancement. Midwives, psychiatric nurses, mental handicap nurses and district nurses now stand a more or less equal chance of getting to the top. This is largely because background discipline and nursing knowledge are becoming less important compared with 'abstract' managerial abilities that transcend local peculiarities and idiosyncrasies. It is increasingly the case that nursing background is required less for its utility than to legitimise the position of managers over a workforce, many of whom may have frustrated professional aspirations. The future might see increased resort to nursing degrees which, apparently, are proving extremely popular, and graduate entrants who will be able to pass through the ranks with indecent haste, ostensibly to gain 'experience' but in reality to obtain the minimum necessary legitimation for their future managerial roles.

So far this has not occurred to any great extent and it may be that graduates will prefer a 'professional' to a 'managerial' model of nursing. They might aim for the increasing number of positions, like those in research, which seem to be outside formal hierarchies, in a 'staff' rather than 'line' relation.[39] At present the grooming of able and not so able elements in the existing labour force has been the only practical alternative. Hence the emphasis placed on management education in the Salmon Report. At each stage the programme of education is more intensive, and particularly at the highest levels its sociological significance is largely aimed at resocialising those who go through it *out of being nurses* and *into being managers.* Such programmes might prove more successful at the highest levels where resources employed in relation to the individual are greatest and where prior commitment is more likely to be assured. At lower levels the effect of a short course has to compete with the influence of institutional factors and a lack of individuals actively wishing to undergo a *rite de passage.*[40]

The logic of such changes is that, especially at the highest levels, there is no particular reason why management of nurses need be carried out by nurses. The further one travels from the ward the less one can talk of 'nursing' or even 'nursing management', but rather management which applies the techniques derived from aspects of capitalist rationality to an area which just happens to be nursing. In the future the new managerial élite may increasingly feel themselves to be managers first and nurses second, or simply managers who are ex-nurses. By contrast, under traditional definitions, the matrons of the traditional élite were always nurses first. Reorganisation carries these tendencies much further. The teaching hospitals are brought firmly within the same management structure which can only narrow the social distance between them and other types of hospitals so characteristic of the traditional system. The managerial content of roles (judging by the 'Grey Book')[41] is much expanded on Salmon. So much so, indeed, that some personnel functions have been hived off to specialised personnel managers. However, against the logic of these changes, nurses have, after much heart searching, been appointed to the new personnel positions.

The inclusion of nurses as full members of the consensus teams at district level and above will create strong pressures towards the adoption of managerial rather than nursing reference groups. For example, the District Nursing Officer is able to include himself or herself in the same group as the District Administrator in order to obtain personal advancement in ways simply not open to a Matron in relation to a Group Secretary. In this the new structure continues and amplifies a feature of all previous structures. To achieve any kind of meaningful equality with other élite groups on the health service, nurses have had to remove themselves from the sphere of clinical decision-making and enter the political sphere. This is a contradiction the medical profession had not yet had to face. It has used its dominance in the clinical sphere as a lever to maintain much of its political power within the reorganised NHS, even though it was only retained by granting, for the first time, formal equality to other groups on the management teams.[42]

The traditional élite always maintained the pretence that in pursuing such a strategy of control outside the clinical sphere they were attempting not merely to further their own sectional interests but to uplift the profession as a whole. To date the newer élite based on the new managerialism has been no different from its predecessors in this respect, though it has been prepared to use more activist methods. Whilst the traditional élite typically suppressed most forms of activity by subordinates, the new élite has on occasions promoted its expression within clearly defined limits. During the Rcns 'Raise the Roof' campaign at the tail end of the 1960s the emergent élite sponsored considerable militancy by student nurses on a pay claim largely designed to widen differentials. This was said to be necessary to attract good recruits and in order to create a new opportunity structure. However the new equality with other élite groups does not entail an uplifting of nursing as a whole. It is an equality won by virtue of the élite's domination over the nursing labour force, an equality which poses no real threat to medical dominance in the clinical sphere.

The New Professionalism?

Such factors have helped to generate considerable disillusion with Salmon at the lower levels of the nursing hierarchy. Amongst trained nurses at ward sister and nursing officer level there has been increasing disquiet at the effects of the full-blooded managerialist solution. 'Inbred attitudes' may play a part, but equally important is the desire of many of these disaffected elements for a clinical solution to their status problem. The Salmon reforms overemphasised the importance of managerial changes in job content to the detriment of clinical changes. It created a formal structure in which power, prestige and remuneration increase with distance from the point of patient contact. Yet with increasing specialisation and advances in medical knowledge nursing administrators are sometimes embarrasingly ignorant of the complexities of the ward situation and this tends to lead ward level staff to resent what appears to them to be a power structure which does not accord with this situation. As Manson argues, there appears to be increasing resentment against interference from senior nursing managers.[43] It is not so much that this interference is new, for the power of the matron at crucial times depended on just that. Nevertheless, a 'custom and practice' of considerable ward-sister autonomy had grown up over the years, which Salmon breached in very important respects.

It is undoubtedly the case that, at these levels, the professional model is being revived. The *ad hoc* growth of postgraduate nurse training, to some extent formalised by the formation of a coordinating Joint Board of Clinical Nursing Studies in 1970, is an important factor behind this revival. Historical figures in nursing history such as Mrs Bedford Fenwick, who was one of the militantly professional nursing reformers, are being 'rehabilitated'.[44] The proposals of the Briggs Report on nurse education pose these questions most directly, not by overturning 'managerialism', but by adding other clinical avenues of advancement.[45] Briggs argues for the ending of the SEN/SRN division in nurse training in favour of a series of modules built around a basic nursing course, followed in Colleges of Nursing independent of service organisations. The major insight of the report is its recognition of nursing diversity, and it represents in many ways a bold attempt to devise a training scheme to cope with this fact. It tries to erase the status distinction between nursing fields that dates from the 1919 Act by making all fields into 'options' and displacing general training from its former preeminent position. Ironically, some of the most vocal opposition to the report has come from nurses in fields previously defined as low status. They seem to be worried that old distinctions will continue in practice, because students will not choose to specialise in 'inferior' options. Under the old system, lack of easy mobility from one sector to another created an almost 'captive' labour force.

The most important proposal of the Briggs Report for the new professionalism is by no means novel: the greater separation of education from service needs. Although not novel, the forces favouring some kind of separation are much greater than in the past. However, implementation would, in the short run at least, be quite costly, in that far greater numbers of auxiliary nurses would have to be recruited to replace student labour. Such a separation between 'clinical' and 'basic' nursing would represent a final break with traditional nursing values. No longer would the performance of basic nursing tasks be seen as noble or worthy in its own right, but as something to be performed only so long as is necessary to learn how to do it. Because more complex tasks take longer to learn than others, more prestige attaches to them. Furthermore, the creation of separate schools would aid the development of an ideology of professionalism. There has, for many years, been a tendency for the 'cosmopolitanism' of the school to come into conflict with the 'localism'[46] of the hospital or service agency. The creation of a group of largely autonomous nurse educators would widen this rift. Under the traditional system, it will be recalled, the authority of the matron seemed to embody both the qualities of the local and the cosmopolitan. The roles of administrator and educator were originally combined, and have subsequently become differentiated.[47]

Because of the economic crisis, Briggs is unlikely to be implemented, except in a diluted form. Nevertheless a general trend of new rifts between managers and clinicians are emerging, as well as the now established rifts between managers and wage workers. These are not hard and fast categories, except at the extreme. The wage worker model fits the nursing auxiliary most, but also fits the large numbers of staff nurses and ward sisters who would not call themselves 'career minded'.[48] As yet, there are few 'pure' clinicians among trained nurses. There are, however, those ward sisters who combine in varying degrees clinical and managerial responsibilities, and those above them in the hierarchy whose responsibilities are almost entirely managerial.

In the mid-1960s managerialism was very much in the ascendent. The new administrative posts suddenly provided an outlet for frustrated elements at ward level. Social mobility on such a scale could only be a once-and-for-all phenomenon. For those passed over, and for new generations of trained staff, career advacement up a non-clinical hierarchy will not be such an open possibility. During the late 1960s there was almost an excess of posts over applicants. In future the situation might be reversed, especially if larger numbers of graduates are recruited. In any case, higher unemployment and the fact that traditional outlets for middle class girls, such as teaching, are becoming much more insecure may mean that nursing will be able to gain the kinds of recruits that élite members have always wanted. If there are not enough non-clinical posts to meet their aspirations it will hardly escape their notice that many present incumbents are people who got there primarily because there was so little competition.

The complex restructuring of the labour force and the decline in traditional forms of leadership are therefore dialectically linked, making the claim by the new managerialists to occupational leadership much weaker. It will not, however, necessarily lead to nurse managers making a complete break from nursing. The resulting vacuum has in part been filled by renewed clinical aspirations by some elements. It has also led to the rapid growth of trade unionism among nurses. Emergent trade union consciousness was closely linked to the restructuring of the labour force. Trade unions were swelled by the growing army of auxiliary and assistant nurses who, whatever their predispositions, were excluded from the professional organisations. They were joined by increasing numbers of rank-and-file trained nurses, who became disenchanted by the careerist ethos of professional associations and their apparent lack of concern with the problems nurses faced as workers. Sometimes this combined with external factors, such as in 1974 when frustration mounted over the effect of successive incomes policies. As a result, it seems almost certain that trade unions have more nurses in membership than the professional associations, even allowing for some degree of joint membership.[49]

In order to understand the complex unfolding of these events it is vital not to lose sight of the changing political economy of health care. Its likely effects on recruitment and the collective bargaining strategy of the nurse managers have already been briefly considered. There are others. In the 1960s managerialism largely emerged in the context of an attempt to effect economies of labour use, but the expansion of the service as a whole was largely taken for granted. In the present context of economic crisis the managerial parameters are fundamentally different. It is one in which we appear to be in transition from a 'welfare' to an 'austerity' capitalism. The prevailing opinion of the government is that we have reached a high water mark in the provision of social services and they are therefore looking to managerial groups to push back the tide even if this means breaching some medical prerogatives. The nurse managers will be forced to play their part in this process. They will have to choose between the manager's responsibility to implement cuts and restrictions in the services and the nurse's desire to maintain and improve them. This situation seems likely to lead to greater conflicts between ward level staff and senior management, as the latter groups are seen to take decisions which lead to a worsening of conditions at ward level. We can see this beginning to happen at present as senior nurse managers play their part by sacking graduating nurses, retiring older nurses early and participating in secret plans with other managers to cut back services in the future.[50] There are also signs that overseas nurses are being victimised at some hospitals, where management have not sought to renew work permits.

Ironically, the situation of economic stringency creates points of alliance between managerialists and clinicians, as well as conflict. The cuts create the possibility of realisation of some professional aspirations, though hardly of the generalised kind that might have followed in the wake of the full implementation of the Briggs Report. The terms of reference of the Royal Commission on the NHS explicitly focus on managerial questions of the 'best' use of labour, In such a context, it will not be surprising if some professional interests press for the delegation of more routine clinical functions from the medical profession. This might centre around the creation of a new grade of nurse based on the American notion of a clinical nurse consultant. This might be based more or less on the Halsbury Report on nurses' pay[51] recommendation of a new higher grade ward sisters, or a redefinition of role for some Nursing Officers.[52] The pressure will be there for the creation of some kind of shorter, clinical hierarchy.[53] A number of 'varieties' have been suggested. Most seem likely to lead to the emergence of rather specialised occupations, like the psychiatric nurse therapists who treat phobias in the community.[54] One might speculate that in the future such groups might well have a tendency to develop a breakaway consciousness, as the claim for professional status might stand a better chance of success through separation from nursing.

In all this talk of clinical nurse consultants and practitioners, two aspects need to be borne in mind. Although many favour some decentralisation of power the problem of how much should be delegated is given little attention. Salmon and reorganisation have created an extremely hierarchical structure into which clinical nurse consultants and practitioners cannot easily be slotted. It is one thing to create a number of specialist roles, with some degree of autonomy from line management, while leaving the main structures of managerialism intact. It is quite another to reorganise nursing work in more fundamental ways on clinical lines. The second aspect of the advocacy of clinical nurse consultancy is its potential divisiveness. While representing advancement for some nurses it may close off opportunities for more interesting work for others. One of the attractive features of nursing as an occupation has been the variety of the workload. Advocates of clinical nurse consultancy seem to wish to cream off the more complex parts of nursing, and deny the right of even the rank-and-file trained nurse to carry out a wide range of duties. One does not have to be an admirer of traditional nursing to recognise that the stratification of nursing work and its fragmentation into basic nursing, clinical nursing and managerialism is against both the interests of the majority of nurses and their need for creative work, and ultimately of a caring service for patients: 'job satisfaction' is being appropriated by a minority of clinicians and managers.

Nurse managers and clinicians, therefore, are at best unable to fight to protect the NHS and, worse, may even stand to gain out of cutbacks. It is not the careerist elements but the ordinary working nurses, trained and untrained, who are beginning the fight to protect their jobs and defend the standards of services. In both these areas it is these groups who are in the front line. There are signs that these nurses, the majority of whom are working-class men and women, are beginning to lay aside their previous social distance from groups like ancillary workers. Only if health workers can act across the rigidly segregated occupational boundaries and reach out into the community, can the present erosion of the NHS be halted, and perhaps be reversed. As the managerial élite abdicates leadership by its complicity with the attack on the NHS, larger numbers of nurses may finally come to believe that they have a greater community of interest with workers at the same approximate level as themselves, than with their own managerial élite.

Acknowledgements

This paper grew out of a discussion and debate with many people. I would especially like to thank Rita Austin, Celia Davies, Bob Dingwall, Andrzej Huczynski, Richard Hyman, Chris Maggs, Sue Pembrey, Dave Towell and fellow members of the Medical Sociology Workshop at the University of Warwick.

Notes

1. Brian Abel-Smith, *A History of the Nursing Profession,* London: Heinemann (1960).
2. Celia Davies, *Continuities in the Development of Hospital Nursing in Britain,* unpublished paper, 1976.
3. In a letter to Mary Jones, quoted by Abel-Smith, op. cit. p. 25.
4. This analysis is similar to that of John and Barbara Ehrenreich, 'Hospital Workers', *Monthly Review* (Jan. 1973), 12-27.
5. F.R. Adams, 'From Association to Union: Professional Organisation of Asylum Attendants, 1869-1919', *British Journal of Sociology,* vol. 20 (1969), pp. 11-26; A. Walk, 'The History of Mental Nursing', *Journal of Mental Science,* 1961, pp. 1-17; E.H. Santos and E. Stainbrook, 'A History of Psychiatric Nursing in the 19th Century: I-II', *Journal of the History of Medicine and Allied Sciences,* 1949, pp. 48-73.
6. Janice Fanning Madden, *The Economics of Sex Discrimination,* Lexington: D.C. Heath (1973), argues that in addition to the existence of sex segregated occupations, there are 'mixed' occupations, in which male workers may adopt a policy of equal pay in order to exclude women workers, by removing the motive for employing them. Psychiatric nursing seems to be such a 'mixed' occupation.

7. Abel-Smith, op. cit., chap. 8.
8. 'Many Years a Matron', in a letter to *The Hospital,* 29 July 1916.
9. Abel-Smith, op. cit., particularly chap. 8.
10. Ibid, pp. 189-90.
11. See the discussion concerning nursing in the USA by Hans O. Mauksch, 'The Organisational Context of Nursing Practice', in Fred Davis (ed.), *The Nursing Profession,* New York: John Wiley (1966), 109-37.
12. Quoted by Jillian MacGuire, *Threshold to Nursing,* London: G. Bell (1969) p. 143.
13. M.E. Baly, *Nursing and Social Change* London: Heinemann (1973), p. 74.
14. *Report of the Committee on Senior Nursing Staff Structure* (Salmon Report), London: HMSO (1966) para 3.17.
15. ibid., para 3.11.
16. Tom Manson, 'Management, the Professions and the Unions: A Social Analysis of Change in the NHS'.
17. National Board for Prices and Incomes (NBPI) Report No. 60, para 47. The recommendations stand in stark contrast to much of the NBPI's advice with regard to other groups of workers where it tended to call for increasing supervision.
18. These were: Mr J. Greene, Chief Male Nurse, Moorhaven Hospital, Ivybridge, South Devon; Miss J. Locke, Matron,Victoria Infirmary, Glasgow; Miss M.B. Powell, Matron of St George's London; Miss E.M. Rees, Matron, Cardiff Royal Infirmary; Miss G.M. Westbrook, Matron of Southmead Hospital, Bristol. All were prominent members of the Rcn.
19. The Salmon Report, op. cit., emphasis added.
20. Once defined by Alan Fox as having only 'one source of authority and one focus of loyalty'. *Industrial Sociology and Industrial Relations,* Research Paper Ho. 6, Royal Commission on Trade Unions and Employers' Associations (London: HMSO, 1966, para 9). However, Fox uses the term in a rather different context to that implied here.
21. The Salmon Report, op. cit., para 3.31, emphasis added.
22. In this it differed from the changes in social work which followed Seebohm. See the analysis by Peter Leonard of changes in the organisation of social work, where there *was* a change from individual autonomy to bureaucracy, in: 'Professionalisation, Community Action and the Growth of Social Service Bureaucracies', in *Professionalisation and Social Change,* The University of Keele, (1973), pp. 103-17.
23. See Muriel Powell in an interview in *Nursing Times,* (1973) pp. 617-8.
24. Christopher Bagley, 'Nursing the Salmon Way', *Health and Social Service Journal,* 1974, pp. 359-60.
25. As, for example, J.W. Paulley, 'Is it too Late to Scrap Salmon?', *Nursing Times,* vol. 67 (1971), pp. 212-3.
26. *Progress on Salmon,* DHSS 1972, para 119.
27. Eve Bendall, 'The Salmon Report: A Tutor's View', *Nursing Times,* vol. 62 (1966), pp. 718-9.
28. Toby Wall and George Hespe, 'The Attitudes of Nurses Towards the Salmon Structure', *Nursing Times,* occasional paper (1972 series).
29. Victor Jupp, 'District Nursing: an Example of Front-Line Organisation', *Nursing Times,* occasional paper (1971 series). The implementation of Salmon in the community followed the recommendations of DHSS: Report of Working Party on Management Structure in the Local Authority Nursing Services (Mayston), 1969.
30. See M. Auld's evidence in 'The Reality of Salmon', *Nursing Mirror,* 27 May 1976, pp. 57-8.

31. NBPI, op. cit., para 67.
32. 'How to Become a Matron', *Nursing Times* (1963), pp. 613-6.
33. K. Jones and R. Sidebotham, *Mental Hospitals at Work,* London: Routledge and Kegan Paul (1962), p. 34.
34. Robert Dingwall, 'Nursing: Towards a Male Dominated Occupation?', *Nursing Times* (1972), pp. 1294-5.
35. 'How to Become a Matron', op. cit.
36. Salmon Report, para 3.32. Or, following Merton, it could be argued that nurses have a 'trained incapacity' for management. See R.K. Merton, *Social Theory and Social Structure,* 1949, pp. 151-60.
37. How to Become a Matron', op. cit. Of course, exactly the opposite case could be put, that many nurses venture into administration because they cannot stand the strain of ward work. In the present context, however, an attempt is being made to get at ideologies rather than truths.
38. R.G.S. Brown and R.W.H. Stones, *The Male Nurse,* London: G. Bell (1973), p. 21. For a good critique see the review by Jeffrey Blum in *Social Science and Medicine* vol. 8 (December 1974), pp. 599-60.
39. E. Bendall and S. Pembrey, 'The Nurse Graduate in the UK: Career Motivation , *International Nursing Review,* vol. 19, no. 1.
40. The present discussion hardly does justice to a highly complex subject which deserves sociological study in its own right. Huczynski has argued that the ability of management education to bring about profound changes of attitude (and behaviour) has been limited by the remoteness of many courses from power realities within the health service and a lack of awareness of the obstacles to change. However, that does not affect the argument presented here which concerns intended rather than actual effects. See A. Huczynski, 'Assessing the Value of NHS Management Courses – Whose Responsibility?', *Nursing Times,* occasional paper (1976 series).
41. *Management Arrangements for the Reorganised NHS,* DHSS 1972, Appendix 3.
42. As Celia Davies notes (in 'Professionals in Organisations: Some Preliminary Observations in Hospital Consultants', *Sociological Review,* 1972, pp. 553-67), the growth in the complexity of the health services although in theory making doctors more dependent on other occupations and lay management, in fact strengthens their power and position because it is they who are legally responsible for patient care.
43. Manson, op. cit.
44. Winifred Hector, *The Work of Mrs. Bedford Fenwick and the Rise of Professional Nursing,* London: RCN (1973).
45. *Report of the Committee on Nursing* (Briggs Report), London: HMSO, 1972)
46. As introduced into occupational sociology by Alvin Gouldner, in 'Cosmopolitans and Locals: Toward an Analysis of Latent Social Roles-I', *Administrative Science Quarterly,* vol. 2 (1957-8), pp. 281-306.
47. This is in marked contrast to the historical development of nursing in the USA. For a discussion of the implications, see William A. Glaser, 'Nursing Leadership and Policy: Some cross-national comparisons' in Fred Davis (ed.), op. cit.
48. The postal survey of the Briggs Report, op. cit. showed that many respondents, trained and untrained, were not actively seeking promotion (Table 45, paras 526-9).
49. 'The response of the Rcn to this fact is to point out that many union members are auxiliary nurses. Given a unified bargaining structure this is hardly relevant. However, it is by no means certain that the professional

associations now have a majority of trained nurses. Significant sections of their membership include students and retired nurses. At the time of writing, the Rcn is in the process of seeking registration as a trade union. Whether in the long run this will mean more than just a formal change in status for instrumental purposes, remains to be seen.

50. National Coordinating Committee against Cuts in the NHS, *NCC Cuts Supplement: Labour and the NHS* (1976).
51. *Report of the Committee of Inquiry into the Pay and Related Conditions of Service of Nurses and Midwives,* London: HMSO (1974).
52. See Rcn: *New Horizons in Clinical Nursing* (1976).
53. See T.A. Kerrane, 'The Clinical Nurse Specialist', *Nursing Mirror* (30 January 1975), pp. 63-5, which asks among other questions: 'Is it true that we are tottering under the weight of administration, while ignoring the desperate need to provide recognition of the clinical nurse?'; Pat M. Ashworth, 'The Clinical Nurse Consultant', *Nursing Times,* 1975, pp. 574-7; Maurice Fenn, Ruby Mungovan, and David Towell, 'Developing the Role of the Unit Nursing Officer', *Nursing Times,* 1975, pp. 262-4.
54. See 'A Symposium on the Psychiatric Nurse Consultant', *Nursing Mirror,* 1975, pp. 46-66 (whole issue).

In his paper Tom Manson draws attention to some of the unintended consequences of the application of an industrial model to the organisation of labour in the British National Health Service. He suggests not only that the model is an industrial one, doubtfully suited to the provision of health care, but that it is specifically derived from profit-making industry and based on capitalist rationality. He examines effects of the increased use of rational management on the attitudes and organisation of ancillary workers. He shows how the introduction of various incentive schemes has led to the development of the consciousness of their common situation among many groups of workers and from that to an increased unionisation and an increased militancy.

He argues that the introduction of the new managerialism has altered the balance of power in the hospital service. In an attempt to increase control over the cost efficiency of the service, a labour organisation has been encouraged which has itself power to challenge the continued running of the service.

Manson sees the consultants as losers in these changes, both from the increased power of the administrators and from the challenge to medical autonomy presented by the now-organised ancillary workers, conscious, especially since the 1973 strike, of their power.

Managerialism has challenged the medical hegemony, a hegemony already being challenged from various quarters which Manson does not discuss here, such as the professional independence accorded to social workers and the increased use of non-medical scientists. Goldie, in a paper earlier in this volume, has shown how limited this challenge may be at present, but it is real nevertheless. One may ask whether Manson is correct when he suggests that the shop stewards' assumption of the right to define what constituted a medical emergency during the 1973 strike was the first overt break in the clinical authority of the doctors. Certainly it was probably the most blatant and the most upsetting, providing a profound challenge to a long-established social order.

M.S.

MANAGEMENT, THE PROFESSIONS AND THE UNIONS: A SOCIAL ANALYSIS OF CHANGE IN THE NATIONAL HEALTH SERVICE[1]

Tom Manson

This paper attempts to locate the development of managerial control in hospitals in the National Health Service within a wider analysis of the problems of health care. The assumption is made that the way in which a health service is planned, delivered and paid for – the organisation of a health service – cannot be seen in isolation from the rest of society, nor from the objectives of those who are involved in the service. At the same time, it is suggested that health service organisation reflects potential and actual social power, since it is the outcome of negotiations, persuasion and sometimes conflict between those who want a form of health care and those who provide it.

Most discussion of the reorganisation of the National Health Service has concentrated on the unification of the various services under the new authorities.[2] While this is an important feature of reorganisation, it is by no means the only one that deserves comment. The new structure was designed to provide the framework within which a more efficient management could plan and control the service. As such the structure was the culmination of a whole series of changes which had begun almost from the inception of the service and which had accelerated throughout the sixties. A number of government reports had pointed out weaknesses. Cogwheel's[3] refers to 'the shortcomings of management arrangements on predominantly medical issues' and argues for a more collective approach to decision-making by consultants when dealing with clinical policy; Salmon created the concept of top management in nursing and implicitly criticised previous nursing management;[4] Report No. 29 of the Prices and Incomes Board drew attention to the need for more efficient management in the service as a whole and in particular to the need for the use of more personnel and work study techniques.[5] Thus in the organisation of medical work, in nursing and in the ancillary grades official reports had claimed that there was a lack of management.

These reports – and there were others, of which one, for instance, covered pharmacy work[6] – were implemented to a greater or lesser degree. Thus before 1974 much of the service had experienced change.

The White Paper on reorganisation made it clear that a major objective was to take such changes on board and to provide the arena within which better management could flourish.[7]

'Cogwheel' was used as an example to show that all levels had experienced some pressure towards improving management. However, the medical profession resisted successfully many of the implications of 'Cogwheel' by claiming that clinical autonomy would be undermined.[8] The real brunt of management change in the hospital service fell therefore on those least able to resist it, and this paper will concentrate on management change amongst the ancillaries and the nurses. The efficient use of resources in the health service has meant that the hospital service has been treated like any other means of production, subject to economies of scale and to the science of management.

Academic work on management in the health service can be divided into two types. First, there is the work closely linked to the creation of the new structure, work designed basically as 'problem solving'. The problem is defined as being the need for greater efficiency in the provision of health care. Solutions have to be fitted into a structure of power and of access to decision-making which is relatively inviolate. Brown, for instance, in one of the most perceptive analyses of the situation, refers to the dominance of the medical profession within the new structure as a 'necessary concession to reality', showing clearly the parameters of control (reality) within which much of the work from Brunel and from Hull is constrained.[9] Given these constraints, one way of accommodating solutions to the established order is to *redefine* power relationships without changing the substance (this is very evident in Rowbottom's work).[10] It is not surprising that the Hull survey of reorganisation, called aptly enough 'New Bottles, Old Wine?'[11] should point to the uncertainties and struggles arising from difficulties in making such concepts as 'planning and monitoring' work.

The main problem with this work is that it does not locate the solutions it advocates within an analysis of the development of the service, in particular within a theory of health care. The need for more efficiency, for money saving, is not seen in relationship to the provision of health care, for health care is seen as the doctors' unassailable province. The relationship between the concept of efficiency and a particular type of medicine is unexplored, but, more importantly, the whole question of the type of medicine provided is not in question. Nor can it be from this perspective.

A further drawback to the 'problem solving' approach is that the effects of the development of management on the service as a whole are not studied in depth. The tendency to skirt the question of power has already been noted. As a result, a detailed analysis of changes in power is impossible. Even if the overall structure of power remains relatively stable, there is room for marginal variation in its distribution. On the one hand, it seems likely that a greater emphasis on management would mean a greater prominence for the managers who would be in a position to limit the discretion of others. On the other hand, a knowledge of the relevant sociological literature on industry would have led researchers to the possibility that demands for centralisation, efficiency and mechanisation, if carried out, might be associated with greater trade union membership, with a consequent increase in some forms of power.[12] Both these features of management change were neglected by those who were involved in the creation of the new structure.

By contrast with this first restricted approach, a second group of academics have taken a wider view of the organisation of health, and have related health organisation to the type of medicine practised. Two examples will suffice in this brief introduction. Powles posits a central paradox in modern medicine: a particular approach, which, following McKeown, he calls 'engineering', is not only producing diminishing returns to scale, but also neglects wide areas of disease.[13] He suggests that there is no questioning of this approach, and indeed recent changes have been based more and more on its application. He sees the relationship between health organisation – high technology, hospital-based – in terms of the structure of power within society and within the system itself. His work is clearly a major advance. However, he fails to analyse the central dilemma of the state in Great Britain faced with the contradictory position of accepting this approach, but finding that the costs escalate without any concrete results. What does the state do, and what are the results? Moreover, what are the effects on the other health workers of an increasing reliance on medical 'engineering', in particular if the workforce is fitted into the technical systems using managerial techniques imported from other 'high technology' industry? If a health factory is created, what about management and the workers?

Another example of this wider approach is given by Robson.[14] Robson sees management change from a different point of view, in terms of the intervention of the market into health care: 'A shift in the balance of power away from doctors who would seek to medicalise the world, towards managers who would market it, is being made with no assessment of the health needs that such structures would be serving.'[15] The cause of this relative decline in professional power has been the state, which through the 'forces of progress' has 'sought a suitable condominium between the professional and local corporate and political interests in the control of health care'.[16] The strength of Robson's analysis is that it has seen a change in power within the service in the light of the interrelation of the medical profession and the state. However, the contradictory position of the state is not noted, nor are the effects of a 'marketing strategy' on other health workers studied. On the other hand, both Powles and Robson do provide insight into wider health care issues, which if supplemented by a detailed study of internal organisation, can explain many developments in the health service.

Management change must be seen as deriving in part from the position of the state with regard to finance, though paradoxically it can also be seen as a reaction to the needs of certain elements of the medical profession. The combination of these factors has created an exercise in efficiency within a framework of medical care to which theories of organisation can be applied.

The compromise of 1948 meant that the state had gained responsibility for financing an institution over which it had very little direct control. Replying to the continual attacks from the BMA, the essence of which were that the proposed National Health Service would undermine clinical autonomy, Bevan repeated again and again that he would allow a great deal of discretion to the profession. In fact, as he later pointed out, he gave them wider discretion, for by removing the cost element from the doctor-patient relationship, the state gave doctors the freedom to prescribe exactly the remedy they considered correct.[17] As Gill put it 'in fact, the introduction of a state financed system of medical care . . . increased even further the degree of functional autonomy enjoyed by the profession.'[18]

This functional autonomy had to be paid for, and Bevan and his officials had little idea what it would cost. Supplementary estimates in February 1949 were nearly 30 per cent above the original 1948 estimate, and thus from the beginning the Treasury was wary of expenditure on health.[19] However, the lack of detailed control over expenditure went further than prescriptions and treatment for individual patients, for at every level in the new service, including the highest level of decision-making, doctors were ensconced, and provided expertise on the basis of which vast sums of money were spent. All the disputes about the control of the health service – whether it should be controlled by local authorities or by the state alone – had fallen by the wayside, and a large measure of control had been given to those who had opposed the creation of the Health Service all along the line.[20] As

Eckstein put it: 'the fact that Parliament drew up such a very skeletal piece of legislation denotes its willingness to abdicate its own influence (and the influence of party) to that of technically specialised groups'.[21]

The state has retained financial control over the service as a whole (which has in practice often meant choosing between plans for expansion provided by different medical advisers) but it has also retained control over certain well-defined areas which few doctors or other professionals considered part of their province. The last two decades have seen an expansion of these areas, mainly at the expense of some nurses who have lost day-to-day control of large aspects of hospital life. It is not surprising therefore that the major struggles over managerialism have taken place between managers and nurses, and the developments within nursing discussed below can be seen as an erosion of nurses' control followed by attempts to regain some of it.

It is important to realise, then, that one of the techniques of financial control was to bring more areas of the service under a more direct control, areas which previously had been subject to the authority of professionals. This technique is part of a more general financial control and might be described as the injection of capitalist rationality into the health service.

There is a large literature on the relationship between technology, investment and work organisation, much of which is derived from the work of Marx.[22] Braverman in particular, traces the development of theories of rational organisation, and of the use of personnel techniques (such as Taylorism) and ties this development to the need for profit.[23] What is important in this context is that most of this theory was developed in private manufacturing industry where there was a clear objective, namely profit. When the state came to look for rational means of controlling the health service, it is not surprising that it used the model of private capitalistic industry, and the techniques derived from this model like work study, separation of skilled and non-skilled elements and in particular the need for management, distinct from the day-to-day running of the organisation and able to function as overall planner and coordinator. Managerialism in the health service can be seen as the use of 'rational' methods derived from private industry, a point Robson makes when he points out that control of the health service 'will be [modelled] on managerial planning evolved for the needs of commercial enterprise in the 1920s'.[24] At the same time this model suits the 'engineering' approach to medicine advocated by much of the medical profession. It is not simply that large hospitals suit the needs of consultants, as Crossman put it;[25] on a more fundamental level, the very organisation of the type of medicine that Powles calls 'engineering' fits in with the organisation of society along capitalist lines. This point was hinted at by Dreitzel when he wrote that 'the Marxist paradigm offers a surprisingly good explanation for certain disastrous aspects of our present organisation of medical care'.[26] Dreitze is arguing, in other words, that much of what is wrong with the organisation of medical care can be traced to the use of capitalist rationality in the identification of illness and its cure. Certainly, in so far as hospital are concerned, some of the resonance of the 'engineering' approach amongst those who plan and control the service is due to the ease with which such concepts as throughput can be applied to the type of medicine practised by those professionals who Powles identifies as 'the purveyors of high technology medicine'.[27] Those areas that can justify themselves in such economic terms are often those which receive the rewards, regardless of their social benefit. This is one explanation for the convergence of the needs of some professionals and those who wish to reap economies of scale through the creation of large hospitals.

The state and elements in the medical profession, then, have combined to create a service where capitalist rationality can be applied. Those areas where it cannot tend to be the areas where the service suffers. The starting point for a detailed analysis of some of the management changes must, therefore, be financial pressure.

From its inception, the National Health Service has been bedevilled by charges that money is being wasted. While the Guillebaud report substantially exonerated the service from these politically motivated charges, a piece of work a couple of years earlier had shown the nature of the problem. The National Health Service is an industry which is highly labour intensive: and in 1955 was becoming increasingly so. Abel-Smith and Titmuss pointed out that costs had increased the most in the hospital service, and a large part of the cost of the hospital service is staff – somewhere between 65 per cent and 75 per cent. Furthermore, 'over three quarters of the total increase of 42,500 in staff is accounted for by more nurses and midwives (21,700) and more hospital domestic and other workers (12,000). The percentage increase in both categories between 1949 and 1953 is substantially in excess of the percentage increase in the number of occupied beds.'[28] This pattern of labour intensity has continued. While in 1949-50 current expenditure was 54 per cent of the total cost of central government services in 1960-1, it had risen to 58 per cent where it remained in 1967.[29] In 1973 there were 153,500 full-time and 86,700 part-time ancillary workers and about 230,000 full-time and part-time nurses.[30] If savings are to be made, therefore, a prime target must be the cost efficiency of manpower, which applies to two groups: the nurses and the ancillaries.

Even if costs had remained totally stable, there would still have been pressure to reduce these given the political climate of the fifties. Abel-Smith and Titmuss showed how labour costs might be reduced by capital expenditure in boilers, laundries, etc. 'The schemes . . . relate to the ancillary departments of hospitals – boiler houses, kitchens, laundries and so forth. The scope for economies in these departments is potentially very substantial.'[31]

Costs however did not remain stable, especially labour costs. Jackson, Turner and Wilkinson in their study *Do Trade Unions Cause Inflation?* point out that there is a great pressure for wages in low productivity areas of the economy (e.g. the National Health Service) to follow those in the high productivity areas.[32] If the crisis is to be circumvented, either wages have to be prevented from rising in line with outside industry (in which case wages remain low) or productivity increases have to be injected. Joan Woodward noted that the rates of pay were low in 1949 in the hospital group she studied,[33] and throughout the fifties wages remained low, but there has been increasing pressure on wages, especially amongst certain groups. It is this pressure, coupled with the growth in costs, that have led to the questioning of the administrative structure of the service, and especially of the methods for controlling the two groups with the greatest numbers – nurses and ancillaries.

The proposals made by Abel-Smith and Titmuss that capital expenditure could save on current expenditure in the hospital service[34] were in fact taken up during the 1960s. In 1960-1, capital expenditure made up 3 per cent of the total cost of central government services; by 1967 this figure had increased to 8 per cent, a substantial real and percentage increase.[35] This increase was due to a large extent to the 'Hospital Plan' produced in 1962. As the BMJ put it: 'The key to Mr Enoch Powell's plan is the District General Hospital.'[36] This plan explicitly took up many of the efficiency arguments, but angled them in terms of the needs of the consultants. It can, however, be seen clearly how mechanisation not only suited the interests of some of the medical profession but also fitted in with a general policy of state intervention to solve its financial problem.

Mechanisation of the various services put immediate pressure on the administrators to use capital equipment more efficiently by the better organisation of human inputs. In the study mentioned above, Joan Woodward's main recommendation was that there should be an increased use of personnel managers, one of whose functions was the fitting of workers to jobs that suited their capabilities.[37] This was in 1949; by the middle sixties the need for a more efficient use of staff to fit in with the increased centralisation and mechanisation was obvious. How this policy would affect the relations between the managers and the professions was not so clear however.

In 1967, the National Board for Prices and Incomes (PIB) published their Report No. 29. While the increased mechanisation had begun a process of management change, its effects had been limited to a small number of experiments. PIB 29 was a watershed, since it claimed that many of the problems faced by the service at the time were due to a management that was not efficient enough. A major spur to efficiency was the use of work study and the use of incentive bonus schemes based on this study. Up to 1967 the terms and conditions of employment of most staff in hospitals was determined wholly through the various National Whitley Councils,[38] after 1967 bonus schemes were increasingly to supplement the national award.[39] For the first time since 1948, therefore, local bargaining could affect the pay packets of many ancillary workers.

To carry through these schemes, however, a different type of authority structure over the ancillaries was essential. The report referred to problems in this area, and also recommended that the number of hospitals administered by each Hospital Management Committee should be increased: 'this would . . . make it easier to secure manpower savings in the manual field through integrating activities and mechanising plant . . . As regards labour management techniques, there is scope for much wider use of work study.'[40] In calling for the rationalisation of the lines of authority in the hospital, for more efficient management, in demanding greater performance from the workers, PIB 29 could not but make an impact on the other elements in the hospital service, a fact the report recognised: 'Such concentration would, of course, have implications for the medical and nursing services which lie outside our reference.'[41]

The introduction of what came to be known as 'bonus schemes' amongst ancillaries began slowly: management change was even slower, and had to wait until April 1974 for its culmination. Bonus schemes were designed to save labour costs: though there were a number of variants, all of them work through the principle that as staffing levels are reduced, those workers remaining should receive a proportion of the labour costs saved by carrying the same amount of work out with less staff. The difficulty arises when the definition of 'the same amount of work' is called into question, and it is here that schemes are allegedly scientific: thus those schemes that work on a simple percentage increase in pay for a similar percentage decrease in staff costs mean that management must be quite clear about the amount expected of the workers in return for their bonus pay. Those schemes based on work study more obviously demand stricter management control systems, since the amount and type of work expected in work time is closely defined: once a scheme is in effect, the targets and methods are set out and the worker will deviate from them at the cost of losing money.

It is, important, therefore, to realise that all bonus schemes stipulate that the control of ward staff be placed in the hands of functional management if the scheme is to work adequately. If a ward sister demands a higher standard of cleanliness than that laid down in the scheme, then the worker who is compelled to carry out this work will lose money. Under a bonus scheme it is highly important that there is a management that lays down the work to be done in a way in which it can be compared with the work of all the other workers in the same section; it is important too that management provides the tools necessary for the job, for without them the worker will again lose money.

The necessity for an increase in the power of functional management was seen early, as was the need to remove ward staff from the direct control of the nursing sisters. The clear recommendation of the Salmon report was that nursing staff should be relieved of non-nursing duties: those non-nursing duties that involved supervising ancillaries should be transferred to administrators.[42] Salmon was of course published before PIB 29 but already by the publication of *Progress on Salmon* problems were arising – in part because of bonus schemes[43] – which will be examined in more detail below.

An obvious possible consequence of bonus schemes was an increase in the power of functional management. Another result was that many groups of workers gained for the first time a sense of group consciousness, and further they gained an awareness of their job: both these factors were an important stimulus to trade union consciousness, and may have contributed to a growth in union membership as well. The agreement between the unions and the management over introduction of schemes contain very clear procedures that must be followed before a bonus scheme is introduced. First of all, the group of workers concerned must be called together to agree (or not as the case may be) to the principle of work study. For agreeing to allow work study to take place, they received £1 per week as a 'lead-in payment'. When the group of workers met together it was often the first time those workers had come together as an identifiable group in the hospital. They were often asked to elect a representative to advise the work study engineers and to liaise between the group and management over the introduction of the scheme. By the time the scheme was in force, the group will have met together at least twice more, and will have become aware that their work has been scrutinised fairly closely. They will have been told in great detail what parts of their work are necessary and what parts are not, they will have been told which tools to use, and what length breaks they can take. In other words, they will have become conscious of all the ramifications of their job and of the need to discuss with management any problems that arose.

The introduction of bonus schemes, together with the general introduction of functional management extended the basis for trade unionism in the service. For some administrators these innovations also made trade unions desirable as channels of information between management and the workers. The membership of NUPE greatly increased in this period, though the union cannot provide figures on where the increases took place. The importance of bonus schemes was seen by one administrator at least. A letter in the *Hospital and Health Services Review,* signed 'non-conformist' read as follows:

> To a considerable extent the Department have themselves to blame for creating a situation which allowed the unions to gain a near stranglehold on hospital ancillary staffs. In implementing the Department's policy for introduction of incentive bonus schemes, management have handed on a plate to unions a wonderful opportunity for massive recruitment – and the offer hasn't been spurned! Membership in sectors where schemes are contemplated has soared to nearly 100%.[44]

Increasingly, since the war particular forms of trade unionism have been accepted by personnel management and by other progressive administrators as being of benefit to the whole organisation.[45] In the National Health Service the abject failure of the local methods of joint consultation – the Joint Consultative Committees (JCC) – culminated in a conviction that joint consultation that was not based on trade unions for its membership could not succeed. As Clegg puts it: 'If joint consultation is to do all that is expected of it, a means must be found of providing responsible and competent representatives who are also in close enough contact with the workers to serve as a means of spreading information amongst them, and of enlisting their cooperation. Representation through the union can give authority to the workers' side.'[46]

The JCC in the area studied by Joan Woodward was already moribund by 1949. Unions cooperated very closely in the introduction of bonus schemes, for instance, and at local level have even paradoxically protected functional management against the professions.[47]

On the other hand, the increase in union membership made the dispute of spring 1973 possible, clearly an unintended consequence of management change, though of course there were other more immediate causes, such as the effect of Heath's pay policy. This dispute can be seen as another watershed, perhaps even more important than PIB 29, since it was during and after this dispute that the latent conflicts within the service began to emerge. Before the impact of this series of selective strikes is discussed, however, it would be wise to refer to the changes that have been taking place in the nursing profession, since they too have had an important part to play in the recent developments in the service.

Mention has already been made of the Salmon report. The effect it had on ancillaries was incidental to the main purpose of its recommendations which was to increase the standard of nursing management, and to provide the framework within which a more rational and effective organisation could develop. The number of nurses had increased dramatically since the beginnings of the service, but the organisation and direction of these nurses had hardly changed. A new structure was called for, which was not designed directly to cut costs – work-study-based bonus schemes were not suggested for nurses – but which was in part a response to the pressures that were common to all to provide a more efficient service.[48] A major objective was to ensure that trained nurses only did work that their training had fitted them for. Under all the principles of rational organisation, it is wasteful to use skilled labour on work that can be carried out by unskilled workers, and therefore it saves money to split work into skilled and unskilled components,[49] with trained staff doing the former. This has clearly been the intention in nursing: ancillaries now are supposed to perform many of the menial tasks once carried out by nurses, whilst an increasing proportion of nursing auxiliaries take many of the more routine nursing duties. By 1973, there were 56, 624 nursing auxiliaries (whole time equivalents)[50] which makes up 21 per cent of the whole nursing profession. In 1949, the figure for 'other nursing staff' was 16 per cent.[51]

While the skill content of the work performed by the trained nurse has increased, paradoxically this has also meant that the span of discretion allowed the nurse has decreased. The intensity of work has increased, while the control over others has decreased. Nursing sisters tend to be much more 'cogs in a wheel' than they had been: not only is there more intrusion from nursing superiors, there is also some intrusion from functional administrators, which at times can cause a good deal of conflict.[52] At the same time, the sister is no longer in formal control of all the staff in 'her' ward – the ancillaries have been alluded to, sometimes training supervisors also intervene in the ward and take control of 'her' students. The trained nurse below the level of the ward sister is more involved in relatively complicated work, but in theory at least, she should be more strictly controlled not by the arbitrary whim of sister, but by the policy of the senior nurses in the district. The extent to which this 'proleterianisation' has taken place is a moot point, but there is no doubt that there is much resentment of the control exercised by senior nurses who 'have not stepped into the ward for years'.[53] The increase in trade unionism amongst nurses, and the 'non-discouragement' by middle-ranking nurses of junior nurses marching and protesting in 1974 owes much to these factors.[54]

The intrusion of functional management into the wards has clearly undermined one aspect of the traditional ward sister's power. Changes from within the profession have had other effects on the organisation of nursing within hospitals. Some of these internal changes have been designed to create a new role for nurses and thus soften the impact of some of the changes noted above. Thus, Michael Carpenter's paper in this volume shows how nurses themselves have initiated reforms and have attempted to provide a new, more clinical role for the middle-ranking nurses, thereby counteracting those 'proletarianising' factors described above.

Anyone visiting hospitals in the summer and autumn of 1973, and enquiring after the effects of the dispute the previous spring would have been told that 'things will never be the same again'. The dispute had a traumatic effect on the service, and brought to a head some of the contradictions created by management change. The most obvious effect was that ancillary workers proved to themselves and to the rest of the service that they had power which, although it could not defeat the government, could, if used at a local level, gain a measure of control over the way the service ran. Workers could close laundries, prevent the running of intra-group transport, close mortuaries: this power could be used again once it was demonstrated that it could work. While there are even now limits to this power over their day-to-day conditions of employment – the Whitley system of National Awards still operates and bonus schemes have been halted by the government's pay policy – there has been a great increase in the day-to-day collective bargaining that goes on. The administration of bonus schemes, the provision of protective clothing, transport to and from work are examples of issues that are increasingly being taken up by stewards and union members: NUPE has reorganised its structure, moreover, in part to encourage this trend.[55] The strike, therefore, increased the power of ancillaries and has encouraged greater bargaining with the administrators.

Management, of course, wanted to understand the lessons of the dispute. A first reaction was to halt the centralisation of the various services – especially the laundries – which had given small groups greater power: a DHSS circular suggested this. It ended, however, with the words: 'NHS management courses for senior staff already include sessions on industrial relations generally.'[56] The implication being of course that senior management should be aware of industrial relations problems. As argued above, this was a long-term trend anyway: all that happened is that the 'progressive' administrators – those who accepted unions and were prepared to bargain with them, to understand and to predict conflict – were strengthened against the old style anti-union hospital secretary. Dyson's report on the strike makes it clear that management will have to continue to bargain and for this reason will have to know with whom they can meet.[57] In these terms, therefore, the dispute served to strengthen the new administrators.

Were these the only effects of the dispute, it would not have been very remarkable. There were further effects which resulted from the effect of any strike on the health service. Most of the bargaining between union and management throughout the dispute concerned the provision of emergency cover. In many cases it was the shop stewards who decided what constitued an emergency: a medical decision. In these negotiations, therefore, stewards began to use their power to make decisions that were essentially medical, and, though it was only a temporary measure, it was the first *overt* break in the power of the doctors. Equally important however, were the arguments used by some of the ancillaries to justify their action. They were in dispute to improve the service, to provide better-paid ancillary workers. If ancillary workers lost out, so would the patients, since ancillaries made, in their view, a major contribution to their welfare. A number of professional made this point when they wrote to the Secretary of State supporting the workers: 'as workers in the NHS we know very well that most ancillary workers are underpaid and that this leads to a chronic shortage of staff which continually affects patient care.'[58] Ancillary workers, therefore, began to see themselves as both in a position to help the patient and justified in doing so.

A final result of the dispute was to introduce to ancillaries the idea of banning private practice. Ancillaries knew as well as anyone where real power lay in the service, so any tactic which hit consultants would have an effect. Many hospitals were forced to shut down private wards during the dispute, and in Portsmouth private practice in the hospitals was banned for months *after* its end. The Secretary of the Charing Cross branch of NUPE also saw the branch's action in the summer of 1974 as a continuation of a tactic they had used in the dispute.[59] But the attack on private practice is, of course, more than a tactic: it is an attack on the dominant group in the service.

The developments in the organisation of ancillary work had been intended to make administrators more important, and their influence had spilt over into the organisation of wards through their control over bonus schemes, and the increase in functional management. It is not, therefore, a difficult argument to sustain that the power of administrators was increasing over day-to-day activities, nor is it impossible to argue that one of the effects of the ancillary workers dispute was to strengthen these tendencies, by encouraging a more 'industrial relations' kind of approach.

In nursing, the increased hierarchy set up in response to the Salmon report was clearly designed to make interventions by senior nursing staff easier in the running of the hospital. In nursing, too, a more 'industrial relations' approach was in evidence as the Royal College of Nursing finally abandoned its opposition to overtime payments and other fringe benefits which had been considered 'unprofessional', and furthermore began to institute a system of representation in hospitals remarkably like a shop stewards system.[60] In ancillary work, and in nursing therefore, the effects of management change had been to increase the power of the administrator, and management change had been associated with a growth in the potential power of unions. Clearly then, any analysis of conflict in the service which ignores the effects of changes in power and the causes of these changes is missing an essential element. The unions are now a force in the health service, whereas, before this period, their influence had been limited.

On a more fundamental level, however, the introduction of management change and its effects raises a number of questions that are relevant to more general theoretical problems. First, questions about professionalisation and the sources of power are important to our argument. In this respect, the relationship between the state and the medical profession has been of crucial importance in the development of the service. But the contradictory position of the state underlines the importance of looking at professionalism not in terms of inherent characteristics, but in terms of the role played by the profession in the wider society and the sphere over which the profession claims jurisdiction. A recent article by Green demonstrates that conflicts between clinicians and administrators cannot be seen as deriving from the nature of professionalism or the nature of bureaucracy, but must be seen in a wider context.[61] One must agree with this, but it still leaves questions unanswered about what this wider context is. This paper suggests that to answer these questions one should look at the complex equation of power between the state and the profession through which the provision of health care is mediated.

A second question that has been raised is how health care itself can be analysed. It is argued here that development of health care can only be understood by linking detailed analysis of the internal organisation of the service with wider social analysis based on an understanding of the state, the professions and the power structure. It is argued also that internal forces within the service have in fact shaken these relationships within society which have created our system of health care. Certainly the medical profession feels less secure than it once did. A recent editorial in *General Practitioner* commented: 'It would be absurd for porters and cooks to tell surgeons when and where they may operate, but this is the kind of situation we are heading towards.'[62] Powerful trade unionism in the health service introduces sources of power and influences over decision-making that are fundamentally different from the old methods. For this reason they provide one link between the detailed internal study and the wider social group.

Understanding trade unionism, however, is no easy matter. One argument in this paper has been that in part at least unions have gained from management change. Many trade unionists realise this: the introduction of bonus schemes was warmly welcomed by the unions and some leaders even saw work study as an antidote to low pay. Furthermore, hospital-based care is supported by the unions since this gives employment to their members. In other words, unions in the health service can easily be drawn into a situation where they merely fight for increased wages within a system of health care which is seen as given.

On the other hand, there is the other element in trade unionism. By organising against the employer at the place of work, by wrestling over decision-making, all unions provide opposition to the unrestricted use of power by the employers. Furthermore, by creating an organisation, they provide an alternative type of power structure to the employers, using a logic which is not that used by the employers. Trade Unions are potential organisations of opposition.[63]

These two contradictory elements, dependence on, yet opposition to, the employer, are present in all unions under capitalism. However, in the health service the picture is complicated by the diffusion of power within the service, as well as the pride most workers have in a service which many of them see as a major advance towards socialism. Furthermore, the unions claim to be the nearest representative there is within the service to those who use the service: as the National Union of Public Employees (NUPE) put it in an advertisement in *Labour Weekly* 'In campaigning for a complete and speedy end to private medicine in the National Health Service NUPE speaks up for the 99 per cent of hospital patients who don't use private beds.'[64] The potential for fundamental change exists within unions, but fully to understand the impact of unions, there must be an understanding of the *contradictory* position they are in.

To conclude, therefore, the relationships between the professions, management and the unions in the health service cannot be seen outside a framework of analysis which places health care in a wider context of the sources and variations of power and the role of the state. Many of the questions arising out of this type of analysis have only been raised in this paper, but they are questions that have to be answered by researchers if the development of health care within this society is to be understood.

Notes

1. The research on which this paper is based was carried out as a joint project by Bob Fryer, Andy Fairclough and myself. At every stage in the production of this paper, my colleagues were involved, and so in a real sense it is a joint effort, and I owe more to their help than is usually covered in disclaimers of this sort. The research was funded from 1973-5 by the National Union of Public Employees (NUPE) and since 1975 by the SSRC. I would like to thank both – but especially NUPE for their help, not only as facilitators but also as sponsors.
2. See for instance F. Stacey, 'Reorganisation of the National Health Service', *Public Administration Bulletin,* December 1973.
3. Joint Working Party on the *Organisation of Medical Work in Hospitals* (HMSO, London, 1967).
4. Ministry of Health, *Report of the Committee on Senior Nursing Staff* (HMSO London, 1967).
5. National Board for Prices and Incomes, Report 29, *The pay and conditions of Manual Workers in Local Authorities, the National Health Service, Gas and Water Supply* (HMSO, London, 1967).
6. DHSS *Report of the Working Party on Hospital Pharmaceutical Service* (HMSO, London, 1970).
7. *National Health Service Reorganisation, England* (HMSO, London 1972).

8. Celia Davies, 'Hospital Consultants and Collective Action' (mimeo).
9. R.G.S. Brown, *The Management of Welfare* (Fontana/Collins, Glasgow 1975), p. 169. It is perhaps unfair to criticise authors for not doing what they had not set out to do. Even so it is argued here that one of the weaknesses of this work (like DHSS, *Management Arrangements for the Reorganised Health Service,* HMSO, London, 1972, strongly influenced by Brunel) is that it is deficient even on its own terms.
10. R. Rowbottom, *Hospital Organisation* (Heinemann, London, 1973).
11. R.G.S. Brown, S. Griffin, S.C. Haywood, *New Bottles: Old Wine?* (Institute for Health Studies University of Hull, Hull, 1975).
12. Two examples will suffice: J. Woodward, *Management and Technology* (HMSO, London, 1958); G.K. Ingham, *Size of Industrial Organisation and Worker Behaviour* (Cambridge U.P., Cambridge 1970). Still the best point of departure however is K. Marx, *Capital,* vol. 1 (Lawrence & Wishart, London 1974), chap. 15, section 8.
13. J. Powles, 'On the Limitations of Modern Medicine', *Science, Medicine and Man,* vol. 1, 1973, pp. 1-30. T. McKeown, for example in 'A historical appraisal of the medical task'in G. McLachlan and T. McKeown (eds.) *Medical History and Medical Care* (Nuffield Provincial Hospital Trust, OUP, 1971).
14. J. Robson, 'The NHS Company Inc.? The social consequence of the professional dominance of the National Health Service', *International Journal of Health Services,* vol. 3, no. 3, 1973, pp. 413-25.
15. Ibid., p. 425.
16. Ibid., p. 422.
17. Aneurin Bevan, *In Place of Fear* (Heinemann, London, 1952).
18. D.G. Gill, 'The British National Health Service: professional determinants of administrative structure' in Cox and Mead (eds.), *A Sociology of Medical Practice* (Collier Macmillan, London, 1975).
19. Harry Eckstein, *Pressure Group Politics: The Case of the British Medical Association* (George Allen and Unwin, London, 1960), p. 136.
20. M. Foot, *Aneurin Bevan* (Paladin, London, 1975) gives a good account of the formation of the NHS, as does Eckstein, op. cit., and Gill, op. cit.
21. Eckstein, op. cit., p. 156.
22. Marx, op. cit., chap. 15.
23. Harry Bravermann, *Labor and Monopoly Capital* (Monthly Review Press, New York, 1974).
24. Robson, op. cit., p. 424.
25. R. Crossman, *A Politician's View of Health Service Planning* (Glasgow, University of Glasgow, 1972).
26. H.P. Dreitzel (ed.), *The Social Organisation of Health* (MacMillan, New York, 1971), p. xi.
27. Powles, op. cit., p. 19.
28. Abel-Smith and Titmuss, *The Cost of the National Health Service in England and Wales* (Cambridge University Press, Cambridge, 1956), p. 33.
29. A.H. Halsey (ed.), *Trends in British Society since 1900* (Macmillan, London, 1972), p. 363.
30. Figures derived from the *Halsbury Report* (HMSO 1974).
31. Abel-Smith & Titmuss, op. cit., p. 133
32. D. Jackson, H.A. Turner, F. Wilkinson, *Do Trade Unions Cause Inflation?* (Cambridge University Press, Cambridge 1975).
33. J. Woodward, *Employment Relations in a Group of Hospitals* (Institute of Hospital Adminstrators, London, 1950).
34. Abel-Smith & Titmuss, op. cit. See Appendix F which is devoted to this subject.

35. Halsey, op. cit., p. 363.
36. *British Medical Journal,* 27 Jan. 1962, p. 238.
37. J. Woodward, op. cit., p. 96.
38. It was in fact *illegal* to pay above nationally agreed rates of pay, one of the few industries where this was the case (if not the only one). See H. Clegg and T.E. Chester, *Wage Policy and the Health Service* (Blackwell, Oxford, 1957).
39. In 1974, 54 per cent of men and 41 per cent of women were participating in bonus schemes; 30 per cent of the workforce in England had rejected bonus schemes. Figures supplied by the employers' side of the Ancillary Staff Council to the staff side.
40. National Board for Prices and Incomes, Report 29, *The Pay and Conditions of Manual Workers in Local Authorities, the National Health Services, Gas and Water Supply* (HMSO, London 1967), p. 21.
41. Ibid., p. 21.
42. DHSS, *Progress on Salmon,* HMSO, pp. 4, 14: 'The Salmon report recommended that nurses should be relieved of non-nursing duties.'
43. Ibid. p. 14: 'the difficulties arising from incentive Bonus Scheme arrangements, particularly those in services for the wards . . . '
44. *Hospital and Health Services Review,* December 1972. It is interesting to note that in the next issue 'non-conformist' was contradicted by a correspondent who signed himself 'conformist'. He wrote: 'Bonus schemes and strikes do not necessarily go together' ibid.: February 1973.
45. Alan Fox, *Industrial Sociology and Industrial Relations,* Research Paper 3, Royal Commission on Trade Unions and Employers' Association (HMSO, London, 1966); for a detailed self-criticism of his former views, see Alan Fox, 'Industrial Relations: A Social Critique of Pluralist Ideology', in J. Child (ed.), *Man and Organisation* (George Allen & Unwin, London, 1973).
46. H.A. Clegg and T.E. Chester, 'Joint Consultation' in *The System of Industrial Relations in Great Britain* (ed.) Allan Flanders and H.A. Clegg (Blackwell, Oxford, 1954).
47. I have been present when a Domestic Supervisor with the full approval of all the domestics, called in the Union to protect her against the Matron who was trying to order domestics to do work they were not supposed to do. The Union made a strong complaint. Interestly enough, the dispute was put down to 'a clash of personalities'. This shows how often those tensions that result from organisational change are attributed to psychological factors or to 'problems of communication'. George E. Wieland and Hilary Leigh (eds.),*Changing Hospitals. A Report on the Hospitals Internal Communications Project* (Tavistock 1971) appear to suggest that many conflicts, which this paper argues are related to the power and interest of various groups, can be solved to a great degree by better communication. The reader will be aware that the author does not agree with this approach.
48. The Salmon report, of course, cannot be attributed *solely* to these pressures: there were others arising from within the service as well. See Michael Carpenter's paper in this volume for a more detailed discussion.
49. The classic discussion of this subject is K. Marx, op. cit., chap. 14. A more recent study of skill in general is H. Bravermann, op. cit.
50. Again these figures are from the Halsbury Report.
51. Halsey (ed.), op. cit., p. 354.
52. See footnote 24.
53. See *Progress on Salmon* for discussion of 'Common fears and misunderstanding' arising out of the Salmon report. The dislike of nursing managers

is certainly 'common'.

54. There has been no study which looks in detail at the nurses dispute. One interesting one is June Morris, 'Nurses fight for themselves and for our health', *Comment,* June 1974. It does not point out, however, that in the early stages, when the RCN was leading the protests, matrons were sending off their juniors to protest with their blessing. As the unions became more involved, however, this soon stopped.
55. Bob Fryer, Andy Fairclough and Tom Manson, *Organisation and Change in the National Union of Public Employees* (NUPE, London, 1974).
56. DHSS Circular DS/301/73. 'Industrial Action by Hospital Ancillary Staff'.
57. R.F. Dyson, *The Ancillary Staff Industrial Action,* Spring 1973 (Leeds Regional Hospital Board, Leeds, 1974).
58. This statement came from twenty four staff at the Department of Psychological Medicine at the Hospital for Sick Children, Great Ormond Street, London. It is referred to in 'Hospital News from NUPE', no. 10, 21 March 1973 (a press handout).
59. This was made clear in a number of meetings prior to the dispute where it was clear that the stewards remembered the effect of a similar ban on private practice in 1973. We have fieldnotes of three of these meetings. See Esther Brookstone, 'Militants and Unions in NHS', *Medicine in Society* vol. 2, no. 1, 1975 for her own view.
60. The RCN also tried to reorganise its structure: see The Tavistock Institute of Human Relations, *An Exploratory Study of the RCN Membership Structure* (Royal College of Nursing, London, 1973).
61. Stephen Green, 'Professional/Bureaucratic Conflict: the case of the medical profession in the National Health Service', *Sociological Review,* vol. 23, no. 1, new series, Feb. 1975.
62. *General Practitioner,* 2 Jan. 1976.
63. This brief paragraph cannot do justice to the theory of trade unionism. A good introduction is: Richard Hyman and Bob Fryer, 'Trade Unions' in John McKinlay (ed.), *Processing People* (Holt, Rinehart and Winston, London, 1975). Also Richard Hyman, *Marxism and the Sociology of Trade Unionism* (Pluto Press, London, 1971).
64. *Labour Weekly,* March, 1976.

Charles Kleymeyer and William Bertrand have contributed what is in many ways an unusual and valuable paper on a mishandled study in Latin America. Over the last few years, there have been a number of reports by sociologists on everyday life in the field and a gradual development of a body of semi-autobiographical literature which, it is to be hoped, will eventually form the raw material for more adequate writings on the nature of the research process. For fairly obvious reasons, though, we still know less about botched projects than about successful ones, although it is possible, as with other areas of enquiry, that deviant cases may be more informative than normal ones. While this paper presents a useful description of the former, its true merit lies in the way that it has subjected failure to a sociological scrutiny. Too often, we only pay lip-service to our discipline, dismissing such failures as the consequence of individual frailty rather than examining the structural situation of the social researcher. The authors show that social scientists may be as guilty of professional *hubris* as the professionals they criticise.

The implications of this paper are not confined to research by Americans in their own dependencies. In some ways, for example, the team described here behaved in an exemplary fashion in the consultation which they did carry out with host country agencies and professionals. The increasing difficulties of research in former colonies which has diverted anthropological interest to the sparsely populated areas of the British Isles has rarely been matched by even this minimal degree of courtesy. The problems of research overcrowding in the North of Scotland and Western Ireland will inevitably provoke demands for outside regulation if we and our international colleagues cannot work more responsibly with local interests.

Similarly, as Kleymeyer and Bertrand note, the lessons of the paper also apply to research in ethnic or working-class communities in our own society. Much is made of consultation and yet it remains unmatched by practical action. It is at least arguable, for example, that some of the difficulties of the CDPs arose from political naïvety and an unwillingness to conciliate official local representatives as striking as the failure of the team described here to conciliate community activists. For both groups, the meaning of consultation was a selective and partial one and both were equally ill-fated.

The authors have presented us with a cautionary tale in the best sense of the word. It stands as both a warning and a prescription for care. Our actions are as amenable to unintended constructions as those of our subjects. The latter is a problem which has been widely debated, the former is as yet barely recognised in any practical sense. Any research provoked by this volume as a whole would do well to remember the self-consciousness of this paper.

R.D.

MISAPPLIED CROSS-CULTURAL RESEARCH: A CASE STUDY OF AN ILL-FATED FAMILY PLANNING RESEARCH PROJECT

Charles D. Kleymeyer and William E. Bertrand

Introduction[1]

A decade after Camelot and its aftermath, social scientists from developed countries have not succeeded in adequately mending their established ways of carrying out applied social science in developing nations (or, for that matter, in less developed or culturally different strata of developed societies). Subjects are becoming less compliant, and problem-oriented studies are still on occasion producing problems rather than solving them.[2] Nevertheless, there is a continuing proliferation of international research efforts falling under the rubric of 'applied social science'. This proliferation has been the result of several mutually supportive trends in the academe and environs. Three of these trends are especially worthy of note. First, a sudden availability of action-specific funds aimed at major social problems created a demand for what was thought to be an existing and prevalent behavioural science expertise in applied matters. Second, because of a dearth of available professionals, major government and foundation funding sources concentrated on producing new experts through scholarship programmes and grants for applied field research. Third, due to continued interest of the developed world in the problems of developing nations, much of the available funds were directed towards such problems, involving both nascent and established professionals in numerous cross-national research projects entailing both 'pure' and 'applied' scientific investigation. This is not to suggest that the problems, explanations and solutions discussed here apply only to cross-national research. As alluded to above, the points to be discussed are also quite relevant to research done across ethnic (and class) boundaries within researchers' own nations.

When dealing with research and development questions which are applied in nature, the concern of funding sources centres frequently on 'directed social change'. It is generally expected that information will be provided either to increase the level of adoption of some practice or technique or to evaluate its acceptance, efficacy or impact. Often, what is asked for is the 'social engineering' of attitudes and behaviour, entailing the manipulation of human beings and the groups they make up.[3] Clearly, the political and ethical implications of such involvement foster some explicit and important questions about both research ethics and research strategies. Related questions arise for applied social scientists from their need and desire to develop methods which are both efficient and socially legitimised for the investigation of present-day social problems.

With the above in mind, we have decided to present a case study taken from a Latin American setting in which the ramifications of these themes were made explicit by a critical set of circumstances and events. The case is one in which North American applied social scientists – two anthropologists and a social psychologist – were involved in an incident with serious and direct implications for a local health programme and for the study population involved. The implications for applied social science were less direct but equally serious.

We want to emphasise from the outset that it is not our intention in this article to place blame on individual actors. The presence or absence of given social conditions and processes make up the critical causal factors associated with the incident. Though some of those social processes were indeed centred in individuals and their actions, such processes and actions did not originate in those individuals but derived from larger historical trends and structural conditions. This is to suggest then that the problem is one of developing and applying a broad research strategy entailing a basically sound, flexible and eclectic approach to a dynamic, complex and always different set of conditions and forces. The task as Gouldner (1970) presents it is one of applying our social science to ourselves *as* we apply it to the 'outside world'.

Our objective in this presentation, then, is to use the case study to make explicit certain problems inherent in applied research and to examine some of their methodological implications and ethical consequences. Others have encountered and dealt with similar difficulties – Adams (1955); O. Lewis (1955); Moore (1967); Selser (1966); Silvert (1965); Tax (1958); Rainwater and Pittman (1967) – and concern has been expressed in many areas of the social sciences regarding these problems – Form (1973); Horowitz (1967); Miller (1965); Portes (1972, 1975); Rodman and Kolodny (1965); Roy and Fliegel (1970). We will attempt to add to this growing literature by presenting a description and analysis of a relevant case.

The Case

The core incident centred around an accusation (which was false, though believed by many and considered seriously by many others) that North American social scientists were involved in a plan to sterilise local children within a government sponsored anti-measles vaccination campaign. This campaign was under the local auspices of an established maternal-childcare programme, developed and administered jointly by a prominent local university and by the City Health Department.

The methodology employed in the case study was the following: The incident itself, including its prelude and aftermath, were observed directly by both authors who were associated with local research and action programmes (having lived and worked in the area for some years) and as such found it desirable to understand a complex social happening which was close to them, even though they were not directly involved in it. The initial method might be called, then, 'fortuitous participant observation'.

As the incident and its related factors took on more and broader importance, a decision was made to design the case study. With little delay, interviews were carried out with health team personnel, city health department officials, *barrio* leaders, local radicals and other persons directly and indirectly involved. The newspapers were gleaned for stories, and informal contacts were subsequently maintained with key persons for many months following the incident. In addition, the better part of a week was spent with one of the North American researchers involved, who came back through town several weeks after the incident. This individual not only answered many questions but voluntarily left a copy of personal field notes which described and analysed the study and the incident. A draft of the present paper was later submitted to each of the three North American researchers for their comments. The same was done with several local professionals (including social scientists) who had first-hand knowledge of the events. As a result of these various reviews, the authors made numerous corrections and additions to the manuscript. In the interest of fairness, every attempt was made and is still being made, to maintain the anonymity of the three researchers. Their institutional affiliation, most of their personal characteristics and, of course, their names have been deliberately omitted from this presentation.

We will begin our treatment of the case with a necessarily abbreviated description of the physical and historical context and the socio-political and socio-economic setting. Then we will describe the prelude to the research project and salient factors concerning that project. Finally we will discuss the incident itself, including its immediate aftermath.

Context and Setting

'Esperanzas' is a slum or poor *barrio* not significantly different from other such settlements which ring major cities throughout Latin America. It had its origin slightly over a decade ago as an illegal squatter settlement which was nipped in the bud by pragmatic landowners and the government who quickly 'urbanised' the threatened area, laying out streets and tiny lots. Esperanzas grew rapidly as the rural poor streamed hopefully into the departmental capital of 'Bolivar'. Bolivar's population itself increased from 638,000 in 1964 to slightly under one million today. The population of Esperanzas rose accordingly – today numbering about 70,000 individuals.

Politically, Esperanzas has a history of being in opposition to the government and to various other outside influences. It is considered by many to be leftist, and there is no mistaking the strength and considerable popularity of the left among the people. The barrio's historical distrust of outsiders includes not only foreigners but outsiders of higher class, status and power (and usually, therefore, of lighter skin). As we shall see, such is particularly true of outsiders who move in and become fixtures in terms of their daily occupations or, at an even higher level, in terms of their place of residence. The occasional visitor is nearly always treated with an abundance of graciousness and hospitality. As is to be expected, it is the more permanent intruder who tends to provoke suspicions.

The most conspicuous outsiders in the barrio at the time the incident was brewing were the three North American social scientists whom we shall discuss shortly. However, a less obvious but in some ways equally problematical group of outsiders was the team of middle-class health professionals from the University and the City Health Department (hereafter called 'the health team'). Even though they were testing a 'progressive' model of health care delivery which differs rather significantly from the norm in terms of its organisation and form of delivery, this team (with one or two important exceptions) consistently relied on traditional forms of social interaction and organisation characteristic of the class, culture and nation in which the team is imbedded. Suffice it to say that the resulting social relations between the health team agents and barrio clients are of a nature generally classified as 'patron-client' by anthropologists and 'vertical' or 'powerful-dependent' by sociologists.

To complete this description of context and setting it is necessary briefly to mention two additional aspects of the general ideological/phenomenological backdrop which impinges upon the behaviour of the people of Esperanzas *vis-à-vis* outsiders, especially those of North American heritage.[4] It almost goes without saying that anti-Americanism and anti-imperialism are strong factors, especially when individuals allow themselves to be identified with the goals and politics of the United States. Another factor is the explosive nature (locally, nationally and internationally) of the topic of population control as well as its close relation, human sexual behaviour, both being topics which played important roles in the incident.

The Prelude

Some four months before the incident itself (the false accusation linking the researchers to an alleged campaign to sterilise barrio children), the future project leader passed through Bolivar on a talent and site search covering several countries and under the auspices of a well-known international organisation. Meanwhile, the university-based institute for which the project leader was working received word from its funding agency that budgets would be cut and that productivity would be looked upon favourably. This news produced a set of predictable tensions and pressures, and the project leader was encouraged to try out some previous ideas concerning applied methodology and family planning (including the cultural acceptability of specific birth control methods). Additional incentives derived from the prospect of publications, further research experience and a month in Latin America. This time span was determined partly by pressures from the funding agency and by competing professional and personal activities.

A few weeks before the study began, the project leader again visited Bolivar, this time to lay the groundwork for the forthcoming month-long investigation. After spending several days making contacts with the University affiliated members of the health team and with a University-based population research centre, the project leader was successful in getting the tentative approval of these two groups for the study (though with some reservations, such as those regarding the small sample size for the home interviews). The City Health Department was approached informally, but the health centre personnel and barrio leaders were not contacted at all.[5] *En route* to another country, the project leader stopped in the national capital and contacted the national planning commission and the local representatives of the US Government funding agency. Thus, the top of the pyramid was well covered, including some persons in the upper echelons of the Bolivar academic structure.

To understand why individuals and institutions in Bolivar gave their approval to the project, we must consider the complex and varied pressures, perceptions and social processes which were at work at the time. First, there were some persons who were genuinely interested in the objectives of the project (though at odds with certain aspects of its approach). Of these persons, some were merely curious, while others saw prospects for direct application of the results. A second general factor in the gaining of approval was that of direct face-to-face persuasion. Skillfully applied and culturally sound social pressures coming from a prestigious professional (as are the majority of visiting North Americans and Europeans, phenomenologically speaking) often prove to be quite effective in the Latin American socio-cultural setting in gaining support for,or compliance with a project, regardless of its practical or scientific merits.

A third factor in gaining approval of the project falls under the general rubric of 'reciprocity and professional politics'. In addition to standard local hospitality, there exists a strong desire to build and maintain relationships with outside sources of funding and other research-related benefits. The resulting 'politics of research' is well understood by some visiting professionals, while others become convinced that it is their personal worth as researchers or problem solvers that elicits such solicitude, hospitality and willing compliance. To expand somewhat on this point, university and government persons and groups frequently perceive visiting professionals – especially those that represent renowned organisations and foundations – as potential sources of goods and services. These range from trips, grants, scholarships, jobs and consulting fees (for themselves, their friends, or their relatives) to free books and publications, invitations to conferences, valuable future contacts, embellishment of personal and/or group reputations and other benefits, both real and imagined. Thus, those numerous local individuals and groups who perceive a broad existing network of institutionalised pay-offs and other valued outcomes, are often hesitant to alienate any sector or representative of that network. In fact, they frequently go out of their way – expending large (sometimes exorbitant) quantities of time and energy – to maintain their inter-institutional and personal contacts and relationships, generally by taking good care of official and unofficial visiting institutional representatives.

A final factor at work in the project's approval was the common one of compliance with or indifference to projects perceived as representing little or no cost or risk. Several local persons involved took a more or less 'who cares?' attitude towards the project due to their interest and involvement in other activities and due to their general assessment that there was nothing to lose by letting the project take place.

The Research Project

A month after the project leader's second short visit, the research team arrived in Bolivar. The next day, a Saturday, they made arrangements to live in an empty house owned and used by the Catholic church in the barrio and immediately left town for the weekend. Monday morning they were back in Bolivar, meeting first with professionals at the university and later in the week with authorities of the City Health Department. At once, obstacles began to arise – ranging from a lack of official communication between the University and the Health Department, to internal conflicts in the target health centre. The Health Department had never been officially informed of the project and thus held off permission to study the health centre for what seemed to them to be an appropriately extended delay – one third of the study period. Finally, the project was approved in its totality. In the meantime, the month had been quickly slipping by, so the two anthropologists had long since moved to the barrio and had promptly begun doing standardised home interviews. When permission came later for the health centre study, the social psychologist joined them.[6]

With the exception of subsequent weekends of rest and travel and short periods of predictable illnesses, the remainder of the month was spent in the barrio collecting data. Interviews and observations were done in the clinic, focusing on the inner workings of that institution. Simultaneously, women were interviewed in their homes concerning their family planning practices, values and attitudes, as well as other topics related to health, health services and procreation. The women were also questioned about their knowledge of the reproductive parts of their bodies (entailing the use of a body chart which rather closely resembles charts used in local family planning courses).

Due to various prior obligations, the three social scientists staggered their departures from the research site. Of an average span of thirty days in Bolivar (counted from the day of arrival until the day of final departure), the mean number of days that each researcher spent in the barrio came to eleven. Though the shortness of this time span may seem extreme and may do damage in the minds of some readers as to the applicability of our chosen case to other situations, we have observed many similarities between this study and others of longer duration.[7]

Furthermore, there were other problematical aspects of the project, in addition to the short amount of time *in situ*, which add to the representativeness of the case. Let us briefly cover several of these problem areas. One aspect – closely related to the extreme limits on time – was the precipitous nature of the researchers' entry into the barrio and of their initiation of data collection. This is to suggest that eleven days of intensive interviewing after two or three months of on-site preparation might have been a suitable time period – at the very least, it would have lessened the chances of misunderstandings and accusations. In contrast, eleven days of intensive data gathering beginning immediately after arrival proved to be risky and counterproductive.[8] Also, the fact that the three unattached researchers lived in a house owned by the local Catholic church led to both ambiguous attributions and later problems because the drug dispensary was in the same house. In addition, one always takes chances when one steps outside the local cultural norms, especially in terms of life-style. An unattached person, for example, renting a room with a family in Esperanzas would be much less likely to arouse suspicion and questioning than three unrelated persons living alone in a temporarily abandoned church house.

Other sources of suspicion and misunderstanding were the researchers' gift-giving and their failure adequately to explain the purpose of their interviews, plus the sensitive content of those interviews. At least one of the researchers innocently and altruistically showered gifts on the barrio children, reportedly even making lists of requests for clothing, school supplies, etc. As a rule in such socio-cultural settings as Esperanzas, children receive presents only from a relative or godparent, so this particular case of gift-giving fell outside any understandable cultural context and was interpreted by many as an attempt to buy off the children. As regards the interviews themselves – especially those in the home – the barrio women reportedly were not adequately briefed either publicly or privately on the nature and purposes of the interviews and thus were left to fill in the blanks, so to speak, with their own interpretations. Finally, the actual content of the interviews was controversial, anxiety-producing and politically volatile. At this moment in Latin America few topics are hotter than the issue of birth control methods and policies.

Two additional and closely related problematic aspects of the research project proved to be serious ones. One was the common practice among US researchers (due to earlier training and dominant contemporary trends in the various professions) of ignoring the possible significance to their research of local, national and international political factors and processes. Some US professionals even argue that such phenomena are 'unscientific' or irrelevant and deliberately do not take political factors into account. Whether this omission be due to innocence or ignorance, it leaves much applied research badly flawed and/or in shambles.

The second, and related, problematic aspect was the previously mentioned failure of the researchers to contact and to gain the approval of the local barrio leadership for the realisation of the project. Perhaps from the distant perspective of the US, those involved felt that by contacting various University people and one sector of the health team they had indeed contacted local authorities. Certainly, in making these contacts they were improving on the practices of many foreign-based research projects of the past. However, they overlooked at least one group – which later turned out to be the key group – the political leaders who make up the barrio's official governing junta.

The Incident Itself

Two days after the final researcher left the barrio for good, a group of barrio leaders came looking for the three North Americans. These leaders had been informed that the City Health Department was going to carry out an anti-measles vaccination campaign in conjunction with the University health team. They had also heard that a team of North American health workers had recently been thrown out of an eastern state of the country for allegedly using a vaccination campaign to sterilise children.[9] This ejection had taken place approximately one week before the three researchers arrived in Bolivar, and at least one of the persons involved reportedly had the same first name as one of the researchers. The sterilisation story had received national and international coverage – front page in the national papers – the accusations being formally retracted several days later (on inner pages). Nevertheless, key persons in the barrio made their own interpretations – in the context described above of problematical relations with the researchers as well as with the health team – and the accusation stuck that the researchers were the same persons who had previously been thrown out of the eastern state.

After four visits in four consecutive days, the group of leaders gave up hope of finding the researchers and went to a prominent barrio priest (a fairly radical and very activist European who is highly trusted and well-liked by the people). Acquainted with the researchers, the priest's reaction to the leaders' accusation was that he thought they were completely wrong, but that if they felt they were right, they should bring him proof. At that, the leaders went to the church house where the three researchers had stayed and returned with a vial marked in English

'STERILE'. The priest explained to them what the word meant in this context, but to no avail. At his request, a highly respected nurse who lives in the barrio (and is also a leftist) explained the different meanings of the word sterile – also to no avail. Finally, the priest took aside the treasurer of the barrio's junta (a man who also happens to be a Sunday school teacher in the parish church) and told him that the people would panic and even more rumours would spread. The treasurer shrugged his shoulders and went on his way.

Soon, young radicals got hold of a portable loud speaker and paraded through the barrio in an automobile shouting, 'Yankee imperialists go home!', 'Our children will be sterilised!', etc. Handbills carrying the same basic messages were distributed, and a local radical paper printed a scathing anti-American editorial likening this 'sterilisation campaign' to US atrocities in Vietnam. Thus, in a loose coalition, the older politicos and the young radicals were consciously or unconsciously, sincerely or opportunistically, playing a catalytic and at times incendiary role. The scandal quickly obtained explosive force. Barrio members began saying they would refuse to have their children vaccinated during the measles campaign, and other clear signs of trouble appeared on the horizon.[10] At that, the health team decided to confront the accusers, before the news media got wind of the incident and things became even worse.

Several intense conversations and meetings were held over a two-day period, culminating in a large meeting which was attended by the barrio leaders, the priest and nurse, the head of the health centre and a doctor and two social workers from the University sector of the health team. At this meeting, the community leaders made three major demands: (1) to receive a sample of the vaccine which would be injected into their children; (2) to receive an official confirmation from the local health authorities that this was a legitimate campaign and that no foreigners were or would be involved; and (3) to be informed in the future of all studies which were planned for the barrio, studies which would be well screened by the health team.

The demands were so reasonable and the health team was so alarmed that all points were accepted forthright. The next day a conservative Bolivar newspaper printed the story of the meeting under the headline, 'Measles Vaccine Does Not Produce Sterility'. Several days later the National Health Ministry felt obliged to put out a nationwide news release assuring the country that the various on-going vaccination campaigns were most definitely not sterilising anyone. By then, things were calmed down in the barrio: apparently people had got what they wanted. The barrio members had their fears of sterilisation assuaged, and the leaders had shown off their concern, responsibility and significance. Perhaps most important of all, they had gone to the mat, so to speak, with the higher-class, higher-power professionals from the health team and had won hands down. Even had they lost in terms of one or all of their demands, they would still have felt victorious because they had forced the powers that be to take them and their constituents into account – at least on this occasion, and perhaps in the future.

The Aftermath

The immediate consequences and future ramifications of the incident were numerous, due in part to the many and changing targets of both the accusations and the barrio's wrath (i.e. the researchers, the health team, outsiders in general, paternalism and imperialism). Fortunately for many of those involved, the incident was well contained and the accusations refuted. These two outcomes were achieved by a combination of the political skills of the health team, the efforts of some respected barrio members and what was either the responsible nature or the ineffectiveness of local press and radio coverage (which was minimal and subdued). Consequently, the progressive health programme survived, the vaccination campaign went off not only on schedule but with no major resistance from the people, and two other North American based research projects in the same barrio were not adversely affected.[11]

For other individuals and groups closer to the scene of action, the consequences suffered – or enjoyed – were more pronounced. Several individuals involved learned valuable lessons, and certain members of the health team were temporarily burned. The North American researchers were left sobered and contrite, and their plans to put the finishing touches on their study, plus the possibilities of a follow-up study, were brought to a quick end. A locally-based foreign researcher found his participation in an on-going, action-oriented research project in the barrio terminated and his longstanding professional relationship with the health team jeopardised. Several other foreign researchers and one foreign research institution were differentially affected by a similar contamination phenomenon.

On the level of group relations, other ramifications of the incident can be noted. The health team subsequently tended to be more careful, meeting more often with barrio leaders, though sometimes only to seek rubber stamping of decisions already arrived at. Nevertheless, such meetings afford an opportunity for the leaders to exert pressure and bring up concerns. All of this just might entail a slight power shift in favour of the barrio, but no changes of a basic nature can be noted in the health team, suggesting that the probability is great that similar problems will resurface in the future (i.e. failure to take the barrio into account followed by barrio leaders applying tactics similar to those chosen during the described incident). As for research projects, especially ones involving foreigners, the health team subsequently demonstrated increased wariness.[12]

In terms of barrio-level ramifications, the leaders temporarily reduced their frustration levels *vis-à-vis* intruding professionals, fulfilled their obligation to serve and protect the barrio and accomplished some individual jockeying within the barrio power structure. The leaders also gained increases in popular support and self-confidence to be utilised in future efforts to ensure that the interests and opinions of the barrio be taken into account. This effect may be temporary, as may be the increased tendency of barrio members to distrust and even fear certain aspects of health services, family planning programmes, research projects and the occasional incursions into their territory of outsiders, be they compatriots or foreigners.

The barrio members were not the only ones to experience at least a temporary increase in their levels of caution. Both nationals and foreigners gained, at least for the time being, an increased respect for the perils of controversial projects such as those which deal with the subject of birth control, or others which entail the taking of blood for research purposes, the use of human subjects in scientific experiments and similar politically and morally sensitive research topics or practices. This aspect has since resurfaced on occasion, e.g. in policy changes. Nevertheless, only future events will reveal the strength and the level of application of this particular lesson, as well as other lessons to be learned from a careful analysis of the described incident.

An Analytical Summary

The incident that we have chosen to describe and analyse is only one of many comparable ones that have occurred in the past few decades. As we have documented, many social scientists have confronted issues of ethical and methodological problems in other cultures. Yet both the particular nature of this case study and its representativeness of that which is presently occurring in various parts of the world has encouraged us to attempt more than an illustrative description of a set of events. Thus, it seems necessary and useful to separate out several primary causal categories which we feel are worth further emphasis and explication.

1. To begin with, the uncontrollable matter of coincidence clearly aggravated the described situation. The fact that the local press carried news of North Americans being accused of sterilising children and that at least one of the names mentioned was the same as that of one of the researchers, helped set the stage for the events which followed.

2. Second, the matter of relevant structural factors of a socio-political nature was of no small importance. The researchers were unavoidably associated with the US, a country whose political and corporate representatives are often in a dominant role *vis-à-vis* nationals of the country where the incident took place. The US is also viewed by some groups of nationals as having imperialistic intentions in its dealings with the country and as being the major source of the country's ills. Furthermore, the paternalistic design, if not the intent, of local health care programmes is characterised by a vertical structure as regards the delivery of services and tends to condition the ways in which an associated group of visiting professionals will be viewed and dealt with. As a result of these structural factors the field workers were perceived by many as outsiders with ulterior motives – as intruders who would have to prove thoroughly the integrity and innocuousness of their motives. Those barrio dwellers who were not so suspicious, were at least open to suggestion and, ultimately, to the accusations. In many social science research endeavours the above factors are present, but even more so in a study which is characterised by high visibility of researchers perceived as belonging to dominant groups, by short exposure to the community under examination and by a delicate, politically volatile subject matter.

3. Social psychological factors, related both to individual behaviour and to cross-cultural misinterpretations of that behaviour, provide the third major explanatory category. Among upper-middle-class North Americans, it is considered appropriate to give gifts, relate directly to children and indulge in gratuitous, unexplained (and difficult to understand) altruistic acts. In a social system where these North Americans are outsiders and power figures (as discussed above) any strange actions can create confusion or can be interpreted as suspicious. Thus, whether due to cross-cultural indifference or ignorance or to simple naïvety, individual actions taken out of their native cultural context can be most problematical within another cultural context. Often, of course, they produce only discomfort or laughter. In other circumstances, the reaction is serious indeed.

Equally difficult for lower-class Latin Americans to interpret is the fact that North American (or any middle- or upper-class) professionals would be willing to reside in the slums. Knowing little of the value (admirable and necessary as it may be) that some branches of the social sciences place on complete immersion in the field setting and on first-hand contact with the social world, the local population applies its own value sets in attempting to explain such strange behaviour. This in turn leads to stories that such persons are secret agents, are reaping huge personal benefits from such sacrifices, and so on. The same phenomenon of cross-cultural misinterpretations led in this case to the researchers' weekend travels being explained by barrio dwellers as trips to the US to make reports and pick up sterilisation serum.

Filling out this third explanatory category are several factors falling within the broad realm of social processes, such as the institutional pressures felt by the researchers, the bilateral desires for professional favour-trading on the part of the health team and the researchers and the barrio members' needs to be taken into account and to assert themselves in the face of familiar irritants. As regards the latter group of persons, we must take into account the broad existing social climate among Third World lower classes which entails not only distrust of outsiders, but also a general alienation from society's institutions and a resentment of past and present exploitation – both economic and academic (especially at the hands of North Americans and other foreigners, and middle- and upper-class nationals).

4. Another general matter which no investigator can afford to overlook is the importance to field research of political factors.[13] These factors change from moment to moment and range from the actions of national governments, to the struggles and bargaining of local politicians, radicals and small-time opportunists. In the present case, the publicised position of the US regarding birth control and the resultant availability of millions of dollars for international work in the area of family planning represented one of those political factors. Local leftist and religious opposition to that stand was another political factor. Widespread anti-American and anti-imperialist sentiment was yet another. The involvement of any social scientist in matters related to population control in developing countries carries with it the risk of political reprisal. It would seem that to ignore this, or to deny it, is to court danger.

5. The final causal category deals with certain factors of an operational nature. Among these were the brief duration of the field work and the precipitous entry into social territories, especially barrio homes, by highly visible outsiders. Also important was the failure to contact

the barrio leaders at any stage of the research and the sometimes problematic relations between the health team and the barrio people. Finally there was the tendency on the part of both the researchers and the health team to rely on an *ad hoc*, crisis-intervention approach to dealing with problems, and the practice of the latter group of giving mere lip-service to the goal of 'community participai

The above five categories and their components entail the more salient and important of the causal factors at play in the incident. For the sake of brevity we have left others out which seem obvious from the analytical parts of our previous description of the case.

Conclusions

Various current political and social changes are converging to force social scientists, especially applied social scientists, to mend our sometimes errant ways.[14] We had best do this sooner rather than later for a variety of reasons, two key ones being the following: (a) because we *should* – in order to play a positive role in people's problems, instead of a negative role or a vacuous one; and (b) because we *must* – in order to maintain any role at all outside of the academe.

In a future work we will present a broad set of measures (e.g. operational, methodological, conceptual, goal-related and ethical) in a discussion of the necessity of field-work reform in cross-cultural settings. Numerous researchers have already touched or concentrated upon one or several such measures in previous works.[15]

It goes without saying, that problems such as those we have discussed in this paper are at one time or another inevitable. Intervention into social problems generates problems: partly because such intervention is usually, in the final analysis, a political action. The fact that applied social science entails problems and politics should not, however, produce an ostrich effect in us, but should force us to make that fact a continual object of study and a component of our methodology.[16] Furthermore, it just might be that current bureaucratic and funding constraints are incompatible with scientific research;[17] and still other problems arise from the conflicting interests of researchers, study population and local and national institutions and pressure groups.[18]

It should be reiterated that this case study has relevance not only for North Americans in Third World countries (as was the case here), but also for *any* social scientists who cross cultural or class boundaries to carry out applied (or 'pure') research. These could be Latin American researchers in the Amazon Basin, Europeans in their own or other countries, or North Americans on Indian reservations or in the inner city.

In closing, we would like to re-emphasise our sociological perspective and our principal goal in this paper. What is called for is a focus on the causal factors not only of a structural but also a social process nature, seeking solutions in the same realms. Since structures and social processes are highly variable and ever changing, such solutions defy rigid formulas. Solutions will be the product of a dynamic methodological and ethical stance which we feel is a necessary condition for the survival of our profession in cross-cultural settings. Also at stake is our effectiveness in the face of monumental world problems, as well as the accuracy of the first and last words of the term 'applied social science'.

Notes

1. The authors would like to thank the following persons for their comments on the contents of this article: Carole Browner, Alejandro Cobo, Cesar Corzantes, Hilda de la Calle, James Greenley, Heliana Kleymeyer, Guillerm Guillermo Llanos, Alejandro Portes, Elias Sevilla Casas, Ronald Schwarz, Jane Trowbridge and the three researchers involved in the case described. During the time the present case study was being carried out, the first author was employed by the Harvard-Cali Program and the International Center for Medical Research; the second author, by the International Center for Medical Health and Tropical Medicine.
2. See, for example, Form (1973); Gouldner (1970); Josephson (1970); Portes (1975); Salmen (1974); Vargas (1971).
3. Mair (1972, p. 287) states this position quite well in her chapter on applied anthropology.
4. For those unfamiliar with Latin America, we might add that the perceptual category 'gringo(a)' and even that of 'norteamericano(a)' has the latent capacity to embrace almost any non-Latin of Western descent, especially those with strange accents, mannerisms, appearances and behavioural styles.
5. According to the project leader, a University official did agree to make all necessary contacts. However, before the research team arrived this official had to leave the country for several months on extended business.
6. Meanwhile, a local psychologist was hired, in a research assistant role, to help interview in the health centre. The project leader insists that this person was a fully-fledged team member (thus balancing out somewhat the heavily foreign and anthropological make-up of the research team). However, this local professional played no role in the research process either before or after data collection, during which time she functioned as an employee of the project. Significantly, she was not perceived locally – either during or after the study or the resulting incident – as a member of the research team.
7. In fact, such hurried studies are common enough in Latin America that they provoke such jokes as the following one which was recently popular in Peru (and perhaps in other countries with only the place names changed). As the story goes, a US academic boarded a plane in Santiago de Chile after a two-week stay, and soon after take-off went forward to speak to the

pilot. When clearance was given, he stuck his head into the cockpit and asked, 'Could you fly low over Peru? I need to add one more chapter to my book.'

One finds additional evidence that such haste is well-known among Latin American researchers and other professionals – they often call such quick-entry-quick-exit research teams 'paracaidistas' (parachuters). A high official in the Bolivar City Health Department had an alternative epithet for such research projects – he classified this particular study as 'Plan Turista' (Tourist Plan). Indicative of the changing climate in Latin America regarding such research is the fact that he said this not in private after the researchers had left the country, but to their faces in a meeting – with a polite smile of course. Yet another observer classified this and similar research projects as examples of 'veraneo academico' (roughly, 'academic summering').

8. Incidentally, the brevity of the study – and the resulting limits on data collection concerning local background and current events – led not only to repercussions during and just after the study period, but to later ones as well. For example, an elementary and sensitive error was made in the introductory comments in the final report – a mistake so glaring in nature as to all but destroy the credibility of the document.
9. Apparently, the local bishop had taken advantage of the North Americans' presence to strike a blow at a prominent family planning programme.
10. What is notable here, of course, is not that the charges were *made*, but that they were – in varying degrees – listened to, believed *and acted upon* by considerable numbers of people.
11. It is interesting to note that both of these latter two projects employ local field workers, have local professionals as co-workers, are focused on relatively non-controversial but relevant topics (immunology and the relation between nutrition and learning), offer highly valued services to participating families (such as medical care, education, food and clothing), and have been in the barrio for several years (not without opposition, but surviving).
12. Nevertheless, research entailing an evaluative component was always viewed by the health team as a potential threat if not simply a nuisance to be dealt with prudently.
13. See Beals (1969); Berreman (1968); Dos Santos (1970); Galtung (1966); Horowitz (1967).
14. See for example, Amaro (1968); Josephson (1970); D. Lewis (1973); Portes (1972); Spiegel and Alicea (1970); Vargus (1971) and an unsigned article in *ASA Footnotes* ('Survey . . . ', 1974). It is interesting to note, that even in the field of applied social science, reforms are generally the result of intense external pressures and of threats to a group's welfare and its survival. One could hope for more (without necessarily expecting it) from such a collection of planners, analysts and problem solvers as we 'applied types' profess to be.
15. Adams (1969); Barnes (1970); Becker (1970); Blair (1969); Clinard and Elder (1965); Cochrane (1971); Denzin (1970); Fals Borda (1970); Foster (1969); Gjessing (1968); Goodenough (1963); Graciarena (1965); Horowitz (1967); Kleymeyer (1973); Maruyama (1974); Peterson (1974); Portes (1972); Roy and Fliegel (1970); Salmen (1974); Sathyamurthy (1973); Spiegel and Alicea (1970); Vargus (1971); Webb (1966); Whyte (1969); Willner (1973).
16. See Gouldner (1970).
17. See Blumer (1967); Bogdan (1975); Clinton (1975); Galliher and

McCartnery (1973); Sjoberg (1967).
18. See Clinton (1975); Rodman and Kolodny (1965).

References

Adams, Richard N. (1955). 'A Nutritional Research Program in Guatemala', in Benjamin D. Paul (ed.), *Health, Culture, and Community: Case Studies of Public Reactions to Health Programs.* New York, Russell Sage Foundation, pp. 435-58.

Adams, Richard (ed.). (1969). *Responsibilities of the Foreign Scholar to the Local Scholarly Community.* New York, Education and World Affairs Publication.

Amaro, Nelson. (1968). *Encuesta sobre el Condicionamiento Socio-Cultural de la Fecundidad en Areas Marginales Urbanas-Metropolitanas, Ladino-Rurales e Indigenas.* Guatemala, ICAPF/IDESAC.

Barnes, J.A. (1970). 'Some Ethical Problems in Modern Fieldwork', in William J. Filstead, *Qualitative Methodology: Firsthand Involvement with the Social World.* Chicago, Markham Publishing Co., pp. 235-51.

Beals, Ralph L. (1969). *Politics of Social Research: An Inquiry Into the Ethics and Responsibilities of Social Science.* Chicago, Aldine.

Becker, Howard S. (1970). 'Whose Side Are We On?', in William J. Filstead, *Qualitative Methodology: Firsthand Involvement with the Social World.* Chicago, Markham Publishing Co., pp. 15-26.

Blair, Calvin P. (1969). 'The Nature of U.S. Interest and Involvement in Guatamala: An American View', in Richard Adams (ed.), *Responsibilities of the Foreign Scholar to the Local Scholarly Community.* New York, Education and World Affairs Publication.

Blumer, Herbert. (1969). 'Threats from Agency-Determined Research', in I.L. Horowitz (ed.), *The Rise and Fall of Project Camelot.* Cambridge: MIT Press, pp. 153-74.

Bogdan, Robert. (1975). 'Conducting Evaluation Research – Integrity Intact', Center on Human Policy, Syracuse University, mimeograph.

Clinard, M.B. and J.W. Elder. (1965). 'Sociology in India', *American Sociological Review,* vol. 30, August. pp. 581-7.

Clinton, Charles A. (1975). 'The Anthropologist as Hired Hand', *Human Organization,* vol. 34, no. 2, Summer, pp. 197-204.

Cochrane, Glynn. (1971). *Development Anthropology.* New York, Oxford University Press.

Denzin, N.R. (1970). 'Who Leads: Sociology or Society?', *American Sociologist,* vol. 5, May, pp. 125-7.

Dos Santos, Theotonio. (1970). 'The Structure of Dependence', *American Economic Review,* vol. 60, May, pp. 231-6.

Etzkowitz, H. (1970). 'Institution Formation Sociology', *American Sociologist,* vol. 5, May, pp. 120-24.

Fals Borda, Orlando. (1970). *Ciencia Propia y Colonialismo Intelectual.* Mexico, Siglo Veintiuno.

Form, William H. (1973). 'Field Problems in Comparative Research: The Politics of Distrust', in Michael Armer and Allen D. Grimshaw (eds.). *Comparative Social Research: Methodological Problems and Strategies.* New York, Wiley, pp. 83-117.

Foster, George M. (1969). *Applied Anthropology*. Boston, Little, Brown & Co.
Galliher, John F. and James L. McCartney. (1973). 'The Influence of Funding Agencies on Juvenile Delinquency Research', *Social Problems*, vol. 21, no. 1, Summer.
Galtung, Johann. (1966). 'Letter to the Ministry of Interior of Chile', in Gregorio Selser, *Espionaje en America Latina: El Pentagono y las Tecnicas Sociologicas*. Buenos Aires: Ediciones Iguazu, pp. 134-45.
Gjessing, Gutorm. (1968). 'The Social Responsibility of the Social Scientist', *Current Anthopology*, vol. 9, pp. 397-402.
Goodenough, Ward. (1963). *Cooperation in Change*. New York, Russell Sage Foundation.
Gouldner, Alvin W. (1970). *The Coming Crisis of Western Sociology*. New York, Basic Books.
Graciarena, Jorge. (1965). 'Algunas Consideraciones sobre la Cooperacion Internacional y el Desarrollo Reciente de la Investigacion Sociologica', *Revista Latinoamericana de Sociologia*, vol. 2, Julio, pp. 231-42.
Horowitz, Irving L. (1967). *The Rise and Fall of Project Camelot*. Cambridge, Mass., MIT Press, 1967.
Josephson, E. (1970). 'Resistance to Community Surveys', *Social Problems*, vol. 18, Summer, pp. 117-29.
Kleymeyer, Charles D. (1973). 'Social Interaction Between Quechua Campesinos and Criollos: An Analytic Description of Power and Dependency, Domination and Defense, in the Southern Sierra of Peru', PhD Dissertation, University of Wisconsin, Madison.
Lewis, Diane. (1973). 'Anthropology and Colonialism', *Current Anthropology*, vol. 14, no. 5, December, pp. 581-602.
Lewis, Oscar. (1955). 'Medicine and Politics in a Mexican Village', in Benjamin D. Paul (ed.), *Health, Culture, and Community: Case Studies of Public Reactions to Health Programs*. New York, Russell Sage Foundation, pp. 403-34.
Mair, Lucy. (1972). *An Introduction to Social Anthropology*. New York, Oxford University Press.
Maruyama, Magoroh. (1974). 'Endogenous Research vs. Delusions of Relevance and Expertise among Exogenous Academics', *Human Organization*, vol. 33, no. 3, Fall, pp. 318-22.
Miller, S.M. (1965). 'Prospects: The Applied Sociology of the Center-City', in Alvin W. Gouldner and S.M. Miller (eds.), *Applied Sociology: Opportunities and Problems*. New York, The Free Press, pp. 441-56.
Peterson, John H. Jr. (1974). 'The Anthropologist as Advocate', *Human Organization*, vol. 33, no. 3, Fall, pp. 311-18.
Portes, Alejandro. (1972). 'Society's Perception of the Sociologist and its Impact on Cross-National Research', *Rural Sociology*, vol. 37, no. 1, March, pp. 27-42; also published as 'Perception of the U.S. Sociologist and its Impact on Cross-National Research', in Michael Armer and Allen D. Grimshaw (eds.). (1973). *Comparative Social Research: Methodological Problems and Strategies*. New York, Wiley, pp. 149-69.
Portes, Alejandro. (1975). 'Trends in International Research Cooperation: The Latin American Case', *The American Sociologist*, vol. 10, pp. 131-40.
Rainwater, Lee and Pittman. David J. (1967). 'Ethical Problems in Studying a Politically Sensitive and Deviant Community', *Social Problems*, vol. 14, pp. 357-66; also in G. McCall and J. Simmons. (1969). *Issues in Participant Observation: A Text and Reader*. Reading, Massachusetts, Addison Wesley Publishing Co., pp. 276-88.
Rodman, H. and R.L. Kolodny. 'Organizational Strains in the Researcher-Practitioner Relationship', in Alvin W. Gouldner and I.M. Miller (eds.). (1965).

Applied Sociology: Opportunties and Problems. New York: The Free Press, pp. 93-113.

Roy, Prodipto and Frederick C. Fliegel. (1970). 'The Conduct of Collaborative Research in Developing Nations: The Insiders and the Outsiders', *International Social Science Journal,* vol. 22, no. 3, pp. 505-23.

Salmen, Lawrence F. (1974). 'Perspectives for Long-Term Co-Sponsored (U.S.-Latin American) Research in Urbanization', Presented at the Seminar on New Directions of Urban Research, Institute of Latin American Studies, University of Texas At Austin, May 1974.

Sathyamurthy, T.V. (1973). 'Social Anthropology in the Political Study of New Nation-States', *Current Anthropology,* vol. 14, no. 5, December, pp. 557-65.

Silvert, Kalman H. (1965). 'American Academic Ethics and Social Research Abroad: The Lesson of Project Camelot', American Universities Field Staff, West Coast South America Series, vol. XII, no. 3, July 1965.

Sjoberg, Gideon. (1967). *Ethics, Politics and Social Research.* Cambridge, Massachusetts, Schenkman.

'Survey Research Problems Getting Worse, Study Shows', *ASA Footnotes* (newsletter of American Sociological Association), vol. 2, no. 5, May 1974, p. 2.

Tax. Sol. (1958). 'The Fox Project', *Human Organization,* vol. 17, pp. 17-19.

Spiegel, Hans B.C. and Victor G. Alicea. 'The Trade-off Strategy in Community Research', in Louis A. Zurcher, Jr. and Charles M. Bonjean (eds.). (1970). *Planned Social Intervention: An Interdisciplinary Anthology.* Scranton, Chandler, pp. 481-92.

Vargus, Brian S. (1971). 'On Sociological Exploitation: Why the Guinea Pig Sometimes Bites', *Social Problems,* vol. 19, no. 2, Fall, pp. 238-48.

Webb, Eugene J., *et al.* (1966). *Unobtrusive Measures: Nonreactive Research in the Social Sciences.* Chicago: Rand McNally.

Whyte, William F. (1969). 'The Role of the U.S. Professor in Developing Countries', *American Sociologist,* vol. 4, February, pp. 19-28.

Willner, Dorothy. (1973). 'Anthropology: Vocation or Commodity?', *Current Anthropology,* vol. 14, no. 5, December, pp. 547-54.

CONTRIBUTORS

William E. Bertrand. Research Fellow, International Center for Medical Research; Tulane University, School of Public Health and Tropical Medicine, New Orleans, La.

Michael Carpenter. Research Fellow, SSRC Industrial Relations Unit, University of Warwick, Coventry.

Mary Ann Elston. Research Fellow, Nuffield Centre for Health Service Studies, University of Leeds.

Eliot Freidson. Professor of Sociology, New York University.

Eugene Gallagher. Professor of Sociology, University of Kentucky.

Nigel Goldie. Lecturer in Sociology, Polytechnic of the South Bank, London.

Gordon Horobin. Assistant Director, Medical Sociology Unit, University of Aberdeen.

Charles D. Kleymeyer. Tinker Foundation Fellow, Centre for Medical Sociology and Health Services Research, University of Wisconsin, Madison.

Tom Manson. Research Fellow, Department of Sociology University of Warwick, Coventry.

Jesús M. de Miguel. Professor of Sociology, Universitat Autonoma de Barcelona, Spain.

Jim McIntosh. Research Fellow, Medical Sociology Unit, University of Aberdeen.

EDITORS

Robert Dingwall. Research Fellow, Socio-Legal Research Centre, University of Oxford.

Christian Heath. Research Fellow, Department of General Practice, University of Manchester.

Margaret Reid. Lecturer, Department of Economic and Social Studies, University of Glasgow.

Margaret Stacey. Professor of Sociology, University of Warwick, Coventry.